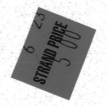

# NO TIME TO DIE

# NO TIME TO DIE
# Liz Tilberis
*with Aimee Lee Ball*

Weidenfeld & Nicolson
LONDON

First published in Great Britain in 1998
by Weidenfeld & Nicolson

Published in association with Little Brown & Co.,
1271 Avenue of Americas, New York, NY 10020, USA

A CIP catalogue record for this book is available
from the British Library

ISBN 0 297 84236 6

Typeset by Selwood Systems Ltd, Midsomer Norton
Printed in Great Britain by
Butler & Tanner Ltd
Frome and London


Weidenfeld & Nicolson

The Orion Publishing Group
Orion House
5 Upper Saint Martin's Lane
London, WC2H 9EA

This book is dedicated with so much love
*to my husband, Andrew,*
*and my sons, Robert and Christopher,*
*who kept me laughing through my darkest moments*

## an absence of foreword

On Friday August 29, 1997, I received voice mail from the assistant to the Princess of Wales. She said that the princess would be delighted to write the foreword to *No Time to Die* and that Diana would call me the following week when she returned to London.

On Saturday August 30 she was involved in the car crash that would kill her hours later.

I could imagine no one else fulfilling this favor, and this page pays tribute to her, my friend Diana, Princess of Wales.

Liz Tilberis
September 1997

# acknowledgments

To Fredrica Friedman for wanting to do this book and for her excellent editorial suggestions; to Jennifer Josephy for guiding me through the complications of book publishing; to Kris Dahl for her never-ending good advice and support; to Aimee Lee Ball, who never wants to hear the name Tilberis again! To Sarah Mower for her endless patience as she traveled through my childhood; to Eve MacSweeney for her patience and energy and teaching me how to line edit! To Annemarie Iverson for all her positive input; to Stephanie Albertson, who runs my life; but most of all to Louisa Terry, without whom none of this book would have been printed!

# NO TIME TO DIE

# 1

IT WAS TO be the most glamorous and celebratory night of my life, a fairy-tale culmination of slavish work and great good fortune. That evening in December 1993, I was at home in New York City, slipping into a floor-length gown of plum-colored panné velvet to greet 250 guests for the sort of soigné party I used to read about in urbane novels and the society pages. Out on the street, the arriving limousines created mini-gridlock and sparked a reverie. I thought of riding the No. 13 bus to my first job as an assistant at British *Vogue* more than twenty years before and the remarkable personal odyssey begun then: becoming the editor of that magazine and now, as a recent arrival to New York from London with my husband, Andrew, and our two sons, editor-in-chief of *Harper's Bazaar*. My mission: to reinvent the flagship magazine of the legendary Hearst Corporation and infuse American fashion publishing with fresh vigor and flair.

The Upper East Side brownstone that we'd rented as our first American home belonged to the director Mike Nichols. It had a triple-height atrium as the main living space and a vast wall of windows overlooking a garden with a koi pond. Everything but the fish was decorated for the holidays. Trailing garlands of pungent spruce hung from the balcony, and dozens of white poinsettias bloomed on every surface—except my grandfather's baby grand piano: The jazz pianist hired for the evening didn't want anything to impede his sound. Two fireplaces were crackling, and on the mantels Santa's elves nestled among branches of flowering quince. White votives and tall tapers were clustered on tabletops laid with vintage linen cloths. I'd personally stood on a high, wobbling ladder to deck the sixteen-foot Douglas fir with tiny feathered robins and glass balls wrapped in bits of old Chinese newspaper and, at the tip, a fat fairy made by my mother just after World War II—not the prettiest girl I'd ever seen, but an important family tradition. Another heirloom had a place of honor near the coat check in the library: a towering Victorian dollhouse, with a dusting of "snow" on its roof and a miniature Christmas tree for its family. Our garden was as vernal as winter allowed, the shrubbery hung with flickering lights and cocooned by a tent suggesting the Arabian Nights, carpeted with kilims and strewn with Moroccan tapestry cushions. Waiters in long white aprons hovered with tempting bite-size spinach tarts and chutney chicken canapés on trays of silver, wood, and slate.

Fashionable New York would gather under my roof that night: friends, business colleagues, and new acquaintances, some to welcome me and show support for *Bazaar*, some to check out the latest in a controversial spate of British imports to head major American magazines. Positioning myself at the French doors near huge sprays of white Casablanca lilies, I began to receive my guests, who were dressed in a stylish spectrum from jeans to tuxedos. Calvin Klein, wearing his signature blazer and T-shirt, is always the first to arrive at any party. "You look wonderful," he said generously, with only a side glance at my plum velvet—by Ralph Lauren, who flashed a huge, appreciative grin when he arrived. Todd Oldham was practically the only other jot of color in the room: New Yorkers wear black by tacit but unanimous consensus, considering it de rigueur for looking sophisticated, sexy, slim, and spotless.

The model Linda Evangelista was seemingly glued to her significant other, the actor Kyle MacLachlan. They were easily the best-looking couple in the room, but Linda deflected my questions about posing together for a cover. "It's the kiss of death," she said. "As soon as any couple do a cover, they break up." Esté Lauder had sent her bodyguard around earlier in the day to determine whether she could manage the stairs and decided against it, but Evelyn and Leonard Lauder were chatting with Revlon chairman Ronald Perelman. There was lots of friendly competition in the room: Donna Karan discussing new lines with Isaac Mizrahi, Philip Miller of Saks Fifth Avenue comparing bottom lines with Gene Pressman of Barneys. Blaine and Robert Trump wearily fielded questions about The Donald, who, as it turned out, was to marry Marla Maples four days later. Nan Kempner, the archetypal socialite, ignored the hors d'oeuvres consumed by Jerome Zipkin, the archetypal society walker, who had brought two large and bizarrely made-up Greek ladies and said to me sotto voce, "There are people in this room who should not be here." I'd hate to think he meant my friend the recently deposed head of Salomon Brothers, John Gutfreund.

I wondered what common interest Knicks coach Pat Riley had with jewelry designer Paloma Picasso. Architect Charles Gwathmey ran into former clients whose modern dream houses he'd designed. The lead singer of Foreigner, Mick Jones, talked music biz with the *Rolling Stone* contingent: editor Jann Wenner and the magazine's former publisher Joe Armstrong, who brought Barbara Walters as a date and the best hostess gift, a string of Christmas lights shaped like cows. Most significant to me were my Hearst bosses: the man who had hired me, magazine division president D. Claeys Bahrenburg; the man who signed my checks, CEO Frank Bennack; and the Big Boss and son of the legendary William Randolph Hearst himself, Randolph Hearst, with his wife, Veronica, impeccably dressed as always in the latest couture. Surveying this stellar crowd with the practiced eye of the professional party-goer were Liz Smith, Neal Travis, and Richard Johnson, taking notes for their gossip columns that would appear in the next day's New York papers.

That evening should have been a blissfully defining moment. Almost two years before, under relentless media scrutiny, I'd been charged with regenerating *Harper's Bazaar* as a fashion force, to rescue it from recent decline and reclaim its preeminence in publishing. Finally the effort was paying off. In April we'd won two Ellies—National Magazine Awards, the Oscars of our own little microcosm, named for the vaguely elephantine statuettes designed by Alexander Calder—and *Bazaar* was garnering kudos from the international fashion community. Hearst had recently taken out full-page congratulatory ads in the *New York Times*, and Christmas was the moment to savor our success, to relax and rejoice in the achievement. It was certainly the best of times.

Except that it was the worst of times. I had cancer. I had *ovarian* cancer, and I was scheduled for surgery the next day—a day that would mean the gift of life or a death sentence. And nobody at that party knew except Andrew and me.

IF ANYONE AT the party had asked me about the previous week, I would have smiled and prattled on about how I'd been so busy closing the March issue—a far cry from the truth. Most of that time was spent in a hazy succession of doctor's appointments, beginning with an innocuous checkup with my gynecologist.

When I'd moved to New York in March 1992, I was invited to a party at Leonard and Evelyn Lauder's art-filled Upper East Side apartment where, after dinner, as a sort of parlor game, the guests made me a fabulous list of the city's "bests": the best dry cleaner, the best fishmonger, the best baker of birthday cakes, the best shops for emergency pantyhose or chilled Chardonnay, the best gynecologist. Dr. Sharon Diamond was nominated top gynecologist, and I took note and went to see her. Tall and slim, with a soft-spoken intelligence, she was close enough to my own age that consulting her felt like having a friend looking out for me. My first visit, soon after the Lauders' party, was uneventful, a routine exam. My records had not yet been transferred from London, but my medical CV was a permanent file in my brain.

In 1978, I'd learned I was infertile, the result of undiagnosed pelvic inflammatory disease that had caused irreparable damage to my fallopian tubes. Desperate to have a child, I'd undergone major surgery in which one ovary and one of my tubes were removed and the other tube cleared. When I failed to get pregnant, I proceeded to nine attempts at in vitro fertilization and repeated use of the fertility drugs Clomid and Pergonal. All the efforts were in vain—I never conceived, and Andrew and I went on to adopt our sons, Robbie and Chris.

As I related this history, Dr. Diamond took a lot of notes but said that I presented an unexceptional and straightforward infertility picture. Since I was no longer interested in getting pregnant, I was told to come back in a year. But I kept putting off that next appointment. On those charts that measure the level of stress in your life, where death of a spouse is 100 and a bad haircut is a 3, I was right up there near the top: establishing myself in a competitive, high-profile job and making a home for my family in a new city, new country, new continent. Typically I'm a sanguine, optimistic person, and I don't often get overwhelmed or depressed, but during the summer of 1993 I was moody and lethargic, begging off almost all social invitations and sleeping for hours on end. Andrew and I both put it down to the move and its lingering toll. We had unfinished business selling our house in London, the boys were undergoing an uneasy acclimation to American schools, and I was in shock over the cost of living in New York where, as a new editor, I was expected to entertain often, and shrimp cost $30 a pound. Even more demanding and difficult were the tasks of hiring people, firing people, and adjusting from the mores and ideology of one magazine empire (Condé Nast, which owns British *Vogue*) to another (*Bazaar*'s corporate parent, Hearst).

On Thanksgiving weekend of 1993, out at the beach house we rented on the eastern end of Long Island, I called the senior staff of *Bazaar* to say, "We've got to sit down and talk on Monday morning." I was fretting about where the magazine was going, and whether we were driving ourselves hard enough and pulling

5

together as a team. Despite our recent awards and success, we'd been a fractious lot, too stressed with the logistics of redesigning the magazine to get to the creative part, the fun. Hindsight now tells me I was casting my own gloom on others. I remember staring out the window that weekend on a dark day that matched my mood and having a flash: *I wonder if I'm sick. Suppose it's cancer.* Such an ominous thought was most unusual for me. I'm not the sort of person who stubs a toe and thinks she's crippled. But something else was going on, and I think, subconsciously, I knew it.

When I came to *Bazaar*, I weighed about 150 pounds, which is practically illegal in our business—even more so in New York than in Europe—and my weight had been the subject of some rude gossip. One newspaper article, one of the kinder ones, called me "bovine." Despite my career in fashion, I never thought of a 23-inch waist as a life goal, and I was always amused by stories from designers who marked their clothes two sizes down when they sold to celebrities. I'd learned to deflect attention from the issue of my weight by mentioning it first—if someone complimented an outfit, I'd retort, "On a good day, I'm a size ten." I *was* quite thin in my twenties and thirties, but ironically, as I was working my way up to the helm of a fashion magazine I started getting chunkier. Andrew attributed it to motherhood—once my children arrived, I turned into Mother Earth—and he grew bigger along with me. There's a picture of the two of us crabbing in Long Island Sound a few years ago: a *huge* Andrew Tilberis and an even *huger* Liz Tilberis. When we walked into the bay, the water level went up. Andrew didn't have the best drinking habits in the world, and I didn't have the best eating habits. I have a limited repertoire in the kitchen, but I love to make classic high-calorie English food like roasts and apple crumble, and one friend jokes that my favorite snack of a Milky Way constitutes all the calcium in my diet.

Under the influence of my slender staff, I'd lost about twenty pounds that first year at *Bazaar*, but now I was starting to gain again. My stomach was bloated and uncomfortable, and I'd been running a low-grade fever. Some of the symptoms reminded me of how I'd felt before being diagnosed with the pelvic inflammatory disease in my early twenties. Back in the city after Thanksgiving, I called for an appointment with my gynecologist as soon as possible. Sharon Diamond was still away for the holiday, so I was examined by her partner, who found some pelvic masses that she thought might be abscesses, a fairly common complication of PID. She prescribed antibiotics and sent me for a vaginal sonogram.

Ultrasound is a painless procedure, but it requires a most ungainly and undignified position, legs splayed, with a probe stuck practically up to your throat. At one point, the technician who was guiding the instrument summoned her colleagues. "Come look at this." As a doctor's daughter, I instinctively know that when the professionals think it's interesting, it's *something*, but no one would say what kind of something, only a confirmed sighting of the masses the doctor had felt.

Dr. Diamond called when she got the ultrasound report. She said that I was not to get alarmed, that this might be a recurrence of my earlier infection, that there might be enough scarring in the abdomen from my tube-clearing surgery to cause these symptoms, but that my history meant I might be at higher risk for ovarian cancer. Infertility is considered to be a significant risk factor for the disease, and a controversial study out of Stanford University the previous year had implicated the use of fertility drugs, particularly for women who never became pregnant. We needed to rule out the possibility of ovarian cancer with a blood test called CA-125, to measure the proteins shed by some cancer cells that induce an immune response.

I did not panic. I thought it was a good sign that Dr. Diamond kept using the word *might*—it all seemed to add up to a definite maybe. I remembered the reassurances that women are always given to allay our fears about cancer. In the face of any anomalous test result, we're constantly reminded, "It's probably nothing." And there is no cancer of any kind in my family, an unusual statistic in itself. I stopped by the doctor's office briefly to have blood drawn for the CA-125 test and scheduled a follow-up appointment to get the results. This time I brought Andrew.

My husband had been skeptical about the need for such a test. I say it sheepishly now, but we had been warned about doctors in America who pad their bills with unnecessary procedures to underwrite their Porsches, as opposed to the National Health Service in Britain, where no money actually changes hands between doctor and patient. When I first told Andrew about Dr. Diamond's concerns, he didn't give much credence to the notion of cancer because in the back of his mind were old warnings from the doctor who'd treated me for infertility that any future pain or bloating could be related to the surgery. I wasn't particularly spooked myself. I was thinking: *Yeah, yeah, this is America. Everyone's hysterical about cancer.*

But by the time we went in, Dr. Diamond had received the results of my CA-125 test. Normal is below 35 parts per milliliter. Mine was over 2,000. She later confessed that she was in a terrible quandary, already troubled and suspicious. There was a dramatic contrast between the pelvic exam of the previous year and this one, and she had her doubts that just an infection could produce those differences. Doctors can be fooled: Something can feel like cancer and not be, or it can feel benign and be cancer. Ovarian tumors often feel hard and irregular and jutting and nodular. That's what she felt when she examined me. But it was three weeks before Christmas. She was trying to spell out what needed to be done and urge me to proceed without delay, without frightening or upsetting me unnecessarily just before the family holidays.

The safe and sensible thing to do, Dr. Diamond advised, was to have a consultation with her friend and colleague Dr. Peter Dottino, head of gynecologic oncology at Mount Sinai Medical Center. Two days later, on Monday, I was in his office. Dottino is an immediately appealing person, the only one of nine siblings to follow his father into medicine, with a demeanor reflecting that hallowed dedication. His voice is streetwise, his body full of kinetic energy, and his handshake numbingly firm. I remember looking at his hands, perhaps to avoid looking at his eyes (which are kind, but they don't lie), thinking: *These are hands that save lives, that may save my life.*

In his tiny office, a cramped mess of paperwork, he pulled a

8

chair out from behind his desk to sit with Andrew and me, our knees almost touching. He wasn't prejudiced by my history or even by my blood test—he had done operations where a pelvic mass and a sky-high CA-125 indeed turned out to be benign abscesses. But when he examined me, he felt certain nodules that meant either severe endometriosis, when part of the uterine lining grows outside the uterus, or cancer. It was impossible to distinguish between the two; I needed an operation either to rule out or rule in cancer.

Dottino's probity is so obvious, his manner so direct and confident, that he completely dispelled any suspicion about a greedy surgeon needlessly cutting people open to make a buck. But his sense of urgency frightened us. "We need to do this tomorrow," he said.

I thought about the possibility that I had cancer (implausible), I thought about the 250 people coming for a party on Thursday (indubitable), and I begged for a few days' respite.

Dottino couldn't believe I was trying to negotiate. "Look, Mrs. Tilberis," he said deliberately, "do you realize what I'm talking about? I don't know if you have ovarian cancer, but if you do, it's serious. What's more important? Saving your life or being the life of the party?"

Andrew and I exchanged a look, realizing the doctor's contempt for *anything* that got in the way of his lifesaving work, especially something as frivolous as a party.

"Will two more days make a difference?" Andrew asked. Dottino sighed and said no.

"Good," said Andrew. "Then we'll have the party."

It made perfect sense to me that the biggest show of my life had to go on—it was my way of keeping things normal as long as possible. But Dr. Dottino made it clear that surgery was imperative. He would operate on Friday and not a day later.


AS FAR AS I'm concerned, Betty Rollin got it wrong. The tele-

9

vision reporter called her courageous, pioneering book about breast cancer *First, You Cry*. But I didn't. There are some life-altering events that hit so hard and fast, you don't cry, and the specter of cancer was like that for me. Andrew and I walked out of Mount Sinai (the same pavilion where Ali MacGraw died in *Love Story*) feeling the heat of that word like a branding iron: CANCER. We said very little. There's nothing to say when you don't know what you're facing, and platitudes are out of the question. With imperfect bravado Andrew kept repeating, "It'll be all right, of course; it'll turn out to be nothing. Goddamn doctors scare the shit out of people."

After only a moment's deliberation, I told Andrew I wanted to go back to the office, to distract myself with work. He understood and, I think, wanted to absorb the information himself. So he kissed me, put me in the hired car waiting at the curb, and walked the few blocks home.

Riding through the crystallized forest that is Central Park after a snowfall, I was as cold as the icicles braided through the trees. All I could think of was my sons: so young, just grammar-school boys. Who would take care of them? Would I see them grow to be men? What careers would they choose? Would their wives be pretty? In the space of a few city blocks, I had morbidly fast-forwarded to unborn grandchildren I might never see. My throat started to close with panic: My husband is an artist, and I had become the breadwinner in the family. If I were sick, how would we provide for ourselves?

Then I got mad: My fucking ovaries had never done me a bit of good, never done what they were supposed to do, and now they were jeopardizing my life. I was outraged, as if I had been sold damaged merchandise and had no recourse with the manufacturer. But finally I started noticing the park, remembering that I was in New York, the best place to be if you had a serious medical problem, and at least now I knew why I had been acting and feeling so foul for the past few months. By the time I got back to the office, I was in control. *No crying*. That's how I handle things—I go into denial overdrive.

Andrew called every hour until I told him to stop—he was interfering with my denial, plus I had important calls to make. Despite my personal crisis, I owed it to Hearst to make sure that *Bazaar* ran smoothly in my absence, which I had been warned by the doctors could be anything up to a month, and I had only three days to organize things. I called my bosses, Claeys Bahrenburg and Frank Bennack, telling both that I was to have exploratory surgery on a suspicious mass. I thought they deserved to know that something serious was in play, and because they are true gentlemen, they responded with total personal support and concern, voicing no business concerns. Claeys offered to do anything possible to make things go smoothly for me at the hospital or for my family at home, and Frank, who has served on hospital boards, called Andrew and volunteered to find me the best second opinions available. No one else at work knew. With the staff, I was purposely vague, using the words "minor procedure" and trying to sound as upbeat as possible. I still half-believed the "minor" part myself. Cloaked in hubris, I couldn't accept that cancer had anything to do with me. I was insulted—how dare such an uninvited foreign entity take up residence in my body? And I called the caterer to check on the shrimp puffs for the party.

I WANT TO say that the night of the party felt like a dream, as I floated in my plum velvet from room to room, listening to the dulcet tones of the piano and the cacophony of exuberant voices. But of course it was a nightmare. I never let my champagne glass stay empty and managed to keep smiling. But inside I felt like Edvard Munch's *The Scream*, artificially tamping down a wordless wail of terror, my anxiety anesthetized by Moët & Chandon. Sometimes I'd catch Andrew's eye, and we'd share the kind of silent, private exchange available to long-married couples. He was smiling too, a big fake smile, knowing that at this time the next day, he'd be waiting for me to come out of surgery, waiting to find out if I would live or die.

I had the passing thought that if this had to be my last hurrah, at least it was just about perfect by my standards: the delightful sounds of music, laughter, and conversation; food for body and soul; everything and everyone looking so beautiful, so happy—even our two Labradors were festooned with seasonal bows. I remember seeing my reflection in the huge mirror over the fireplace, the blurred vision of the festivities going on behind me, like Audrey Hepburn in *Sabrina* watching the splendid patrician gala at a Long Island estate from the treetops near her home in the chauffeur's quarters. But I was no chauffeur's daughter. I surveyed the crowd, thinking: *Is this me? Is this my home? Is this my life?* All night long, I vacillated between a moment of exhilaration and a jolt back to reality, stung by the reminder of what awaited me the next day.

Much of the evening's badinage is lost to me now. I was grateful for any momentary amusement, like Joe Armstrong, a Texan by birth, trying to convince Andrew that he wasn't a real American until he owned cowboy boots. I know I buzzed about, making sure everyone's glass was filled, warning people not to spoil the dogs with too many treats, making a fuss over the children who came with their parents—miniature fashion plates in their serious, starchy Sunday-best clothes. Then I saw Grace Coddington, who was getting ready to leave. Grace and I have known each other since I started working with her at British *Vogue* in 1969 and have shared everything that's happened in our lives since. We'd traveled halfway around the world together, and toasted more New Year's Eves than either of us cared to remember. She was the first friend to hold our first son. Even though she was now creative director of American *Vogue*, *Bazaar*'s greatest rival, we were intimate friends, with a bond that couldn't be jeopardized by professional competition. It was midnight, the hour when I was supposed to heed the presurgical instructions about having nothing more to eat or drink, and I knew I had to put down my champagne flute. I panicked: no more alcohol-induced numbness.

Just as Grace started to say, "Liz, everything was so . . ." I pulled her into the corridor outside the kitchen, grabbing her arm so hard I could feel her bones.

"Oh, God, Grace," I blurted out, "they think I have ovarian cancer, and they're operating on me tomorrow."

Her face froze, and her body slackened. I thought she was going to faint, and I grabbed on even tighter, drawing so close that her red hair grazed my cheek and whispering, "You can't let on. But what am I going to do?"

She didn't speak—she didn't have to. As we stood clutching each other for a moment, she was too stunned to summon up any platitude intended to convey comfort. The terrible look on her face made me realize the import of my words, and began to chip away at my wall of denial. It was the fear reflected in her eyes, more than any internalized dread on my part, that made me linger downstairs with the detritus of the party, forestalling sleep, long after the last guest had kissed the air behind both my ears and departed.

But even then, even with the shock I saw in my best friend's reaction, with the attentive caresses of my husband, and with the ominous cautionary language of doctors ringing in my ears, I didn't believe, I *wouldn't* believe, that I really had cancer.

# 2

I WAS THE village idiot about ovarian cancer when I went in for my surgery. But I could barely remember my own name that day: I had a horrific hangover.

Early that Friday morning, December 17—no coffee, tea, aspirin, or "hair of the dog that bit me" allowed, and no breakfast—Andrew and I went to a carol service at the boys' school. It was so peaceful to sit there with all the proud parents, listening to the choir sing "Silent Night." I couldn't have planned for a better antidote to the anxiety of the past several days. Most of my time had been taken up with blood tests, X-rays, more blood tests, electrocardiograms, more blood tests, CAT scans, and, for a change, blood tests. When I wasn't baring my veins, I was wrapping presents for the boys and stowing them under the Christmas tree. Robbie was twelve and Chris just eight, so they'd been told only that I was going to the hospital for some tests. I staunchly refused to address the sobering legal ramifications of the surgery that would determine whether I lived or died. I didn't write any "In the event of my death . . ."

letters, not to my sons, my parents, or my lawyer. I didn't even have a will drawn up.

We'd ordered a car service to drive us to the hospital, and Andrew stayed until I was admitted and had relinquished my clothes for a green gown, foam slippers, and cotton cap. But he couldn't bear to wait out the surgery in the "family room" where half the people would be crying and the other half trying to be nice to him. I held him with a vise grip as he kissed me and said "See you soon," but there were no tears. Then he went to a bar and tried to calm himself. When beer didn't work, he switched to scotch, but no matter how much he poured down his throat, the worry kept him sober.

I was stone cold sober myself and would have killed for a Valium (or a hit over the head with a hammer) as I was wheeled miles and miles through the bowels of the hospital to a holding bay outside the OR. I felt so sorry for all the sick people on gurneys lining the corridor. A nurse handed me a consent form, granting Peter Dottino permission to take out any part of me he found necessary to remove. I hardly recognized him in surgical scrubs, with only his serious eyes visible over the rim of a mask. In the two days since we'd met, he'd gone from addressing me as "Mrs. Tilberis" to "Liz," or sometimes "kiddo," and I called him "Peter." My last words to him before the anesthesia began to take effect were, "I know I don't have cancer." He clutched my arm and said, "I hope you're right."

I HAD CANCER. Stage III ovarian cancer.

The operation, which was to have taken two hours, stretched to four, while Andrew went back and forth to the post-op room, terrified that I had died. When I woke up in the recovery room, Peter was standing over my bed saying, "You're going to make it, kid; we caught it in time." Still in his surgical greens, he had found Andrew to report in reassuring terms that I was alive and the prognosis was good. He had removed my remaining ovary and fallopian

15

tube, my uterus, part of my colon (rejoining the pieces with those magic hands so I thankfully didn't need a colostomy) and the omentum, the apron of fat that covers the intestines. (I deeply believe it is the absence of this padding that allows me to stay slim, but Peter assures me this is a figment of my imagination.)

"Did you get it all?" is the first question you think of when you wake up from cancer surgery, but it turns out that's not even the intent with ovarian cancer, which tends to be spread around in little Rice Krispy-size particles. The largest tumors are removed in a process called "debulking," and the goal is to leave no tumor larger than two centimeters. Anything smaller than that can be eradicated by chemotherapy.

Confronted with a diagnosis that could no longer be dodged, my denial was supplanted in one part of my brain by a degree of equanimity, the calm of the inevitable. But I was in the most excruciating pain imaginable. Searing and incessant, it felt as though the operation were still taking place, without anesthesia—actually, it felt as though I were being cut in half with a chainsaw—and I didn't care that the surgery had been successful if success meant such agony. Fortunately the pain people came to my rescue. That's what they called themselves, those angels in green who stood at the foot of my bed and said, "We're from the pain department." What they provided was bliss: PCA, or patient-controlled analgesic, which is a nice way of saying morphine on demand. There was a button attached to a pump on my IV pole, regulated by a tiny computer. One push, and the sweet relief was immediate. No waiting for a nurse, no relatives yelling "Give her the shot!" like the Shirley MacLaine character in *Terms of Endearment*.

I was in recovery for one day, my midriff wrapped in a thick, sticky bandage; I was terribly parched but forbidden to drink—it's curious how something like thirst can seem even more of an ordeal than pain. Sucking on glycerine-soaked sponge lollipops was like receiving manna from heaven. The next morning, I was moved to my own room in the oldest part of the hospital, a ward run by a fierce group of enormous women—well-trained nurses but frighteningly impersonal—and the indignity of being vulnerably depen-

16

dent began to hit home. There was a little bell to summon help, but the nurses didn't come right to the room—they answered on an intercom, which could be heard in every other room. So I'd press the bell to say, "I'm going to be sick," and they'd say, "I didn't hear you," and by that time I'd be throwing up. Or I'd say, "I need a nurse, please," and they'd bellow back, "Why?" and I'd have to announce to all the world that I required a bedpan. Not only did everyone on the ward hear my entreaties, I heard all of theirs too. It was so demeaning and inefficient, turning adults into three-year-olds, but I tried not to be a bother, not to cry wolf. I'm sure the nurses were overworked and underpaid, but their agenda was not about kindness, it was about getting a day's work done.

On Christmas Day, I was running a fever, and there was some concern that my wound was infected. It turned out I was allergic to the bandages—just my sensitive English skin fighting with the plastic—and as soon as they were removed, my temp went down. But the battle-ax of a head nurse would not let my children in to visit. Andrew could see the boys' eyes filling with tears, and he went ballistic. Dr. Dottino had gone out of town for the holiday, so Andrew went barreling down the corridors until he found the vice-chairman of the department, a solemn and imposing figure named Dr. Carmel Cohen. "Listen," Andrew bellowed, "you'd better tell this insensitive old cow that we're going in to see my wife even if I have to use force." I suppose it was his flash point, releasing the tension of the past days. He knew it would have been unbearable for me and for the children not to see one another that day, and Andrew is a man who knows when a war's worth fighting. The boys got in.

It was Andrew, of course, who had the task of getting our sons through the emotional shock of seeing me in the hospital. He hesitated to use the word "cancer," but he didn't want to lie, rightly anticipating that they might hear the word from somebody else, so he told them the doctor had taken care of the problem, and although it might be scary to see me that way, I'd be home soon. Kids are remarkably resilient about such information, and with the help of my magic morphine button, I was able to grin and bear it

17

for their brief visit. Andrew had tried to organize a proper Christmas dinner for them at home, but he didn't want to be bothered making a whole turkey. So he got a cooked breast and some dark meat from a caterer nearby and assembled a sort of half-assed holiday bird on the platter. The boys were not impressed, regaling me with stories about the "rent-a-turkey."

*I* wasn't allowed to eat anything myself until I started making what are delicately called "bowel sounds"—unfortunately, Claeys Bahrenburg arrived just in time for that. I had few visitors, since almost no one knew I was in the hospital and so many people were out of town that holiday week. Andrew came morning, noon, and night, but only for ten minutes (he is not good at bedside vigil), bringing treats to tempt my sluggish appetite. One day he bought out McDonald's, which I can recommend to anybody in the hospital—the smell alone brought on an absolutely Pavlovian response. We got into the habit of sneaking the boys in every day for five minutes—they were extremely well behaved and managed to avoid Nurse Ratched. I was visited by doctors all day long, and grew accustomed to waking up with a group of white coats standing around the bed, pulling down the sheets, and whipping up my nightie. They were always trying to drape some shred of decorum over a few inches of my private parts, but it hardly seemed to matter—all modesty had gone out the window. I did nearly faint when I saw my scar, held together with clamps and staples like Frankenstein's zombie. The resident who took them out was an empathetic woman who promised it wouldn't hurt, but sat on my bed and cried with worry about a friend of hers who had done many cycles of the same fertility drugs I'd taken.

By the time I left the hospital two weeks later, it seemed like the entire world knew about me, at least in my own media microcosm where gossip travels like the common cold. None of it was malicious—we are, after all, in the information business. Claeys Bahrenburg had informed my creative director, Fabien Baron, who went to Paris and told Karl Lagerfeld, whose salon at Chanel is Mission Control for fashion industry news. My health bulletins were bruited around various water coolers on both sides of the

Atlantic. It was really an open secret, my privacy honored by a tacit gentlemen's agreement, until I was "outed" by an industry newssheet, *Folio*, which ran the announcement of my illness framed in a box on the front page. It was nice that *Bazaar* was called "one of the hottest magazines in the business," but it did preempt my decision to go public, and the item was roundly denounced by other columnists the next day. (In the *New York Post*, I was wedged in between tidbits on Mia Farrow and Lorena Bobbitt.)

Almost everyone else was kind and solicitous. Much of South America must have been pillaged for the bouquets that were delivered almost hourly to the house. The fax machine in our library spewed out a constant stream of thermal paper filled with messages, drawings, newspaper clippings, and good wishes. Delicious care packages showed up on our doorstep from a gourmet market called E.A.T. that's notorious for its $16 grilled cheese sandwiches—Evelyn Lauder had decided to supervise my diet. Another friend sent a dish we called hamburger pie because it reminded the boys of shepherd's pie in Britain, only with macaroni substituted for mashed potatoes. Donna Karan and Adrienne Vittadini made Jewish and Italian versions of chicken soup, and Daryl Hannah, who was on the cover of *Bazaar* that month, sent brownies over with a young man on a bicycle who turned out to be John F. Kennedy, Jr. (Andrew didn't recognize him and was quite rude—it was early Sunday morning.)

I'd been warned not to climb too many stairs after surgery, so we decided to put a bed in the ground-floor dining room for afternoon siestas. I hated it—couldn't get used to napping where I should have been carving roast beef, and anyway the dogs kept jumping on top of me. Mostly I'd sit in a big blue-and-white striped chair, snuggling under the cream-colored cashmere blanket sent by Ricky and Ralph Lauren, taking calls and receiving guests. My mother called every day, mostly to say, "I wish I could be there," but she was overwhelmed with caring for my father, who'd already sunk too far into aged ill health to recognize me, let alone travel to see me. He was never told that I had cancer—we decided

19

to spare him the worry. But my brother, Grant, and his wife, Sarah, both physicians, visited from Britain. We ordered Chinese takeout and talked about cancer survivors they knew who had gone on to have babies, or climb Mount Everest, or fly to the moon. Their well-intended pep talks gave the impression that the only thing a cancer survivor couldn't do was cure cancer.

Shortly after I got home from the hospital, Andrew answered a ringing phone, and an English voice said, "Hello, it's Diana."

"Diana who?" he asked, rather bluntly.

"It's Diana Windsor," she said, and Andrew handed the phone to me with a broad smile, mouthing the word "princess."

That was the first of many calls from the Princess of Wales to check on my health, and the reality that I will never hear that voice again is hard for me to accept. The princess first came into my life in 1987, when I was editor-in-chief of British *Vogue*, and we kept in regular touch until her tragic car crash in August 1997. We were friends, but I was her royal subject—curtsying when I saw her and addressing her as "ma'am." (It was always tricky to get the curtsy in before she came forward for a kiss.) A call to someone recuperating from cancer surgery isn't easy for anyone to make, but the princess wasn't scared of illness, and was well known in Britain for her low-key dedication to visiting the sick and needy, when she always seemed graciously relaxed. Her conversations with me were full of appropriate sympathy but also bits of small talk and scandal, about who was pregnant and who was fat, who was dating whom and who was divorcing whom in the circle of Britons we knew in common. She was always so warm and open, it was easy to suspend formalities and just dish. (I once complimented the Chanel shoes I'd seen her wearing, with their insignia of interlocking *cs*. "I think of them as Charles and Camilla," she said mischievously.) While we were talking, we were interrupted by call-waiting beeps, which I chose to ignore. (Wouldn't you, if the Princess of Wales had called?) Finally she asked, "What *is* that?" and when I explained, her laughter had a hint of relief. "In England," she said, "it would be MI5"—the Ministry of Intelligence, Her Majesty's Secret

Service, equivalent of the FBI, who were rumored to have bugged the princess's phone.

Unlike Diana, most people don't have a clue how to react when someone has cancer. They're unsure whether to acknowledge the illness or ignore it, whether they're close enough to send good wishes or being intrusive by making contact. Some people are melodramatic in expressing their feelings, and others can't even begin to find words. The worst for me were the letters from people who had lost a loved one. I'm sure they were meant to make me feel lucky to be alive, and I *did* feel lucky, but I couldn't take on the burden of a stranger's sadness. Andrew screened the mail every morning, keeping back anything he thought would be bad for morale. I wouldn't presume to lay down any rules of cancer etiquette, but the most meaningful notes I got were the ones that made me feel less like an invalid, offering a report from the outside world, a hint of scandal, some gossip from the couture, a bit of humor. Even if I couldn't eat half the things that people sent or was too tired to take a call, the thoughtfulness they showed was heartening. There is nothing like being sick to make you realize how people feel about you. As the new year approached, the house was still decorated from the party, the cancer was gone, my family was starting to smile again, and I was full of hope. I felt cocooned, protected and loved.

THEN I HAD to look in the mirror.

I work in an industry that is acutely judgmental about appearance, and we spend a lot of time observing one another. It's our business to notice everything: clothes, shoes, hair, makeup, weight. It's information-gathering of an essential kind for our trade. Editors are the first "real" women to try out ideas from the catwalks of the fashion shows that we transmit in due course to the reader. We love doing it and seeing how others do it. The ability to scrutinize women and assess their looks is a prime unwritten qualification for being a fashion editor. There's a bitchy side to such analysis, of

21

course, and evidence of ineptitude is great fun. In 1995 I was thrilled to receive a prestigious Matrix award from New York Women in Communications, but I was completely distracted at the luncheon ceremony, where the entire dais of middle-aged media stars, from Oprah Winfrey to fellow honoree Cokie Roberts, was a sea of red. I wanted to drag them all out into the sunlight with a mirror and say, "Don't you see how bright colors reflect on the face and make you look thick and harsh unless you're twenty-two?" And we're always making fun of the meteorologist on CNN, blending into the weather map because the lime green or hot pink of a Canadian cold front matches her neon jacket. Like any insular group—ballerinas with their leotards and legwarmers, bankers with their rep ties and pinstripes—editors have their own specific rules about what's acceptable, and to outsiders we can seem merciless in our observations. But it's absolutely legitimate professional behavior.

Factor in the "ambassadorial" part of my job: Publicity is vital to getting the magazine noticed, mentioned, and sold. I can't stay behind the scenes. When I arrived at *Bazaar*, I became the subject of a kind of chronic surveillance: What would I do? Whom would I hire and fire? How would my *Bazaar* differ from its previous incarnations, as well as from the competition? As interest escalated, it was important that I be photographed at fashion shows, be seen at charity benefits, host dinner parties, be interviewed on TV, and generally put my face forward to promote the magazine. It didn't even occur to me to change tack when I got cancer. In fact, my illness and the issues surrounding it were to propel me further into the public eye than ever before.

But I was about to start chemotherapy and enter a whole new world of technical jargon I had never hoped to have the opportunity to master.


CHEMO USUALLY CONSISTS of several drugs combined in a "cocktail" so the tumor doesn't become resistant to a single component.

The genesis of chemotherapy dates back to World War II, when doctors examining sailors who'd been exposed to mustard gas found that most of their white blood cells had been destroyed. Since leukemia is a type of cancer that produces too many white blood cells, medical research began to focus on the possibility of using chemicals intentionally to kill cancer cells. Today standard "conditioning" for ovarian cancer includes cisplatin, a distant relative of the platinum used in fine jewelry, which binds with the DNA of the cancer cells to prevent them from dividing and reproducing. (One of the side effects of chemotherapy is akin to heavy-metal poisoning.) Usually, chemo is given in six to eight sessions spaced three to four weeks apart. But Peter Dottino had just written a protocol, or blueprint, for a different regime based on a recent theory called "dose intensification," in which the treatment is accelerated to just nine weeks. In a more compressed time, the drugs seemed to attack the cancer faster, stronger, better. He got me into the program.

Shortly after the new year, I went back to the dismal citadel of Mount Sinai. The chemo drugs came in a powdered form that had to be ordered from the pharmacy and liquefied in an IV bag. But first I was hydrated to protect my kidneys, which meant taking in gallons of water through the IV and making constant trips to the bathroom. (The nurse put an upside-down "hat" in the toilet and waited for me to pee a certain amount.) When chemotherapy is given by IV, the caustic chemicals can burn and scar the skin. So, in a short, one-time-only surgical procedure for which I was blessedly put to sleep, a port catheter was inserted beneath the skin just below my collarbone, leading directly into a major artery and dumping the drugs quickly into my bloodstream. It looks like a mesh basin that attaches to the needle where the drugs are dripped in. I didn't have to get stabbed repeatedly in veins and in vain. The nurse could hook me up with one swift poke, as I held my breath against the piercing of tender skin.

Living with a port cath under the skin seemed a small sacrifice for my lifeline to chemo—it just meant no spaghetti straps or bustiers, and once a month it had to be flushed clean. Everything to do with this device had to be scrupulously sterile because it led to an artery near the heart. I was given a little ID card for my wallet in case I was in an accident and a paramedic tried to access it under nonsterile conditions. Once I burned my hand cooking, and the emergency room personnel backed away from my port cath like it was a plague sore. (Some studies have shown the value of intraperitoneal chemo, which delivers the drugs right to the belly rather than making them travel through the bloodstream, but the studies have not included the newest drugs used to treat ovarian cancer.)

ASIDE FROM THE initial puncture, chemo for my type of cancer is not painful, but it's miserable. Each session lasted about twenty-four hours, and I'd sleep that night with the medicine dripping every few seconds, the whir of the monitor a kind of demonic lullaby. I usually went into the hospital on a Sunday, and on Monday I would sit at home, unable to move even if my shoes had been on fire. I threw up only once, when I foolishly persuaded the resident on duty to make the drip go faster than usual, but it was like being seasick all the time: Even if I wasn't vomiting, I was nauseated, unable to eat or even be around food, with a constant metallic taste in my mouth.

Since the platinum was destroying the white blood cells that normally protect against infection, I was given daily subcutaneous shots of a "fertilizer" called gross cell stimulating factor that makes the body start producing white cells again. I was told I could learn to inject myself in the leg, but I couldn't bear the idea and paid an enormous amount of money to have a nurse come to my house at five o'clock to do it for several days in a row. I had to wear white paper masks everywhere—to the office, the movies, the stores. Andrew thought I presented something of an image problem and refused to accompany me to Bloomingdale's, but I never even noticed people staring, I was so excited to be shopping.

After the first few treatments, as predicted, I started losing my hair and had to make some decisions about my appearance. I'd been wearing my hair in a shoulder-length bob for as long as I could remember, but Didier Malige, my great friend, master hairstylist, and companion of Grace Coddington, said, "It's going to fall out anyway, so why not go short?" I've since learned that this is wise counsel for any woman about to undergo chemotherapy— it's somehow more traumatic to see long strands of hair spiraling down the bathroom drain than to deal with the hair issue straightaway and accept the temporary idea of wigs.

People have always made a big deal out of the fact that my hair is white, in an industry—and a culture—where youth and beauty are revered, and women (not to mention covert numbers of men) pay thousands of dollars to keep the color of their youth. I started to go white at twenty-seven, and it never bothered me. What *would* have bothered me was hours sacrificed to sitting in salons with foul-smelling poultices on my scalp. Yes, I edit a magazine that runs regular features on carefully tawnied or boldly peroxided hair fashions, but I don't have the attention span for it myself. Once, looking at photographs in the art department, somebody referred to an older gray-haired model as "La Grise." I said, "If she's La Grise, then I'm La Blanche," and the name stuck.

Everyone seemed to like my new gamine haircut, but I wasn't sure I was ready to give up my signature long hair and decided to have my wig made long—it could always be cut. But I didn't know how to find something natural-looking, something that wouldn't shout "Wig!" or, worse, "Halloween!" Tonne Goodman, my fashion director, solved that brilliantly. Where do you see the best wigs in close-up and not even know what you're looking at? In the movies. Tonne's mother-in-law, Piedy, is married to the director Sidney Lumet, and Tonne found out that the best theatrical wigmaker was another British ex-pat named Paul Huntley. He agreed to see me even though he does not take private clients, and I walked into a studio filled with styrofoam heads labeled "Julia Roberts," "Glenn Close," and the names of dozens of other film stars. By this time, five weeks into chemo, I had no hair at all, so I brought photographs to show what I looked like before chemo.

25

Paul's wigs are made on a base of fine mesh tulle, so delicate that you can see the scalp through it. Mine was so convincing that even people who knew me well didn't realize I'd lost my hair. I put it on, and there I was, me with my shoulder-length bob again. I was back!

Andrew reasoned that if we could find a way of making the wig a joke, it would ease the boys over the shock of seeing me bald. When the wig was sitting on its pompous little purple stand, it looked like the one Laurence Olivier had worn in *Henry V,* so Andrew dubbed it "Larry," and once it had a name, it seemed much less threatening. Although I had Larry in residence on top of my head, I also lost eyelashes, eyebrows, pubic hair, underarm hair, and the hair on my legs—everything except my "mustache," a bitter cosmetic irony. The eyes may be the windows to the soul, but it is the brows and lashes that really contribute to facial expression, and my face was naked and static, incapable of expressing a raised brow of surprise or a grimace of disbelief, like that of a Hollywood space alien. I found people staring at me rather more intently to ascertain my mood. If I'd lacked vanity about my prematurely white hair, I was incredibly vain about my eyelashes—my special endowment from the family gene pool—and I couldn't even wear false ones because my lids were too red and puffy. I learned to deal with "chemo face": drawing in eyebrows with a charcoal pencil, emphasizing my lips, toning down the classic chemo flush.

Larry was a love/hate affair. Whenever Christopher had a friend coming to the house, I'd ask, "Is this a wig playdate or a non-wig playdate? Do you want me to look like the Mummy that used to be?" He didn't like Larry but usually voted for it over the extraterrestrial look. Chris was just beginning to establish his peer group in New York and didn't want to bring any secondary problems into his friendship-making. Sometimes I wore scarves, but they made me feel like women in the 1950s who tried to cover their curlers when they went shopping. Baseball caps were more me and made the kids happy. The trouble with a wig is that you can't feel if the wind blows it out of place, so people were patting down my hair all the time. The damned thing seemed to have a will of its own, often misbehaving in public. We'd be waiting in line at a restaurant or movie, and Robbie would lunge at my head. On the job, when I was out with my editors, I'd feel a friendly *Bazaar* hand reach out and smooth my hair back into place without saying a word.

I decided to wear a wig to work, rather than throwing my chemo head in people's faces, as if asking for attention or sympathy. But as I got stronger and felt better, I became more defiant about leaving Larry off. So I was nearly bald. So what? If I could live with it, so could everyone else. Andrew encouraged my temerity, even when I had what was virtually a buzz cut. "I don't give a fuck about anybody else," he said. "I'm saying it looks great. It's sleek and smart. It's even sexy. Just do it!"

It's hard to keep your spirits up when you're looking and feeling so drained, but you cannot allow yourself to dwell on the side effects of chemo or regard it as poison. It's a life force, an ally, a weapon, a friend. I had to focus on a deadline, if not to be well, then at least to make a public appearance for the sake of the magazine, so everyone could see that, as in the words of Mark Twain, the rumors of my demise had been greatly exaggerated. Several months earlier, before cancer had entered the equation, my creative director, Fabien Baron, had been selected for an award from the Council of Fashion Designers of America, and I had promised to introduce him at the glamorous awards ceremony at Lincoln Center in February. I intended to keep that promise. But I'd lost thirty pounds, and my flesh was hanging in folds. It was one of the few times in my life when I could look in my closet and honestly say, "I have nothing to wear."

I was so fortunate to have access to the most creative problem-solvers. It's not every woman in my condition who could rely on Julia Roberts's wigmaker or call Ralph Lauren for another velvet dress, this time in blue and several sizes smaller than the Christmas plum. I didn't attempt the cocktail party or gala dinner, going directly backstage, where I shared a dressing room with k.d. lang and Rosie O'Donnell, but I was so weak, I could barely apply lipstick, let alone join in the girl talk. It was Miuccia Prada who gave me a much needed shot of adrenaline: She saw me sitting in the wings, clasped my hand very tightly, and said, "I went through the same thing many years ago." I managed to carry the hefty award onstage, and Fabien started to cry when he took the winged statuette from my shaking hands. As I tried to remain upright, I didn't say anything memorable, but Fabien was extremely generous about my part in his winning of the award.

A week later I was to be given an award of my own at a benefit for the Lighthouse, a charity for the blind and a meaningful occasion for me as the daughter of an eye surgeon. Calvin Klein sent over some long slip-dresses with Zack Carr, the design director of the company, and a lovely-looking woman named Carolyn Bessette, who worked in public relations. Zack wanted me to wear silver satin, but I was afraid that all the ridges and bumps from my still-healing scars would show through. Carolyn read my feelings completely. "Stop putting her in the silver things," she instructed. "She doesn't have the confidence right now. Let her wear black!" She knew that a familiar "uniform" would be more comfortable and would cover a multitude of sins. That kind of mettle has probably served her well in her marriage to John F. Kennedy, Jr.

I arrived at the Waldorf-Astoria Hotel to find 600 people who wanted to shake my hand and say hello. I don't think anybody realized how frail I was—I suppose I just seemed thin—but I was so shaky I had to sit down in the middle of conversations. Philip Miller, chairman of Saks Fifth Avenue, introduced me and somehow I managed to climb up to the podium, slowly and steadily, feeling 1,200 eyes boring into the back of my head. I made a brief speech, describing the time my parents traveled behind the Iron Curtain to Czechoslovakia, where my father was given two dozen pairs of soft contact lenses by a professor in Prague who was eager to smuggle out the formula. I talked about a career in which the visual is all-important. And no one seemed to know that my chic little beaded bolero jacket was covering my port catheter.

Another public appearance I made was at a party to celebrate the opening of Richard Avedon's exhibition "Evidence 1944–

1994" at the Whitney Museum of American Art in March. *Bazaar* hosted the event, as Avedon had been the star photographer for the magazine from 1945 to 1966 and had revolutionized fashion photography by introducing movement into his pictures. It was another celebrity-filled evening, and at Avedon's insistence, he and I (in Larry) made our rounds to each table to say hello to the many guests: Calvin and Kelly Klein, Donna Karan, Gianni Versace, Raquel Welch, Brooke Shields, Naomi Campbell, Isaac Mizrahi. As I became rather tired trying to keep up with Dick's energy, I felt something on my back and realized it was Andrew's hand, making sure that I was still standing, whereupon Dick exclaimed, "Oh, Liz, I totally forgot that you are going through chemo!"

AS IF CHEMOTHERAPY wasn't enough of a jolt, welcome to instant menopause. Everything dried up, including my sex drive, an all-too-common occurrence in the wake of cancer, as I learned when I started looking into the subject. "Going through chemo and menopause together is like a holocaust experience," says Dr. Carolyn Runowicz, director of gynecologic oncology at Montefiore Medical Center in New York City, who got the patient's perspective firsthand when she was diagnosed with breast cancer herself. "You're trying to survive, not trying to live, and sex takes a back seat." Even when you put chemo behind you, your insides are not the same after a hysterectomy. Surgical menopause can be much more severe than when it happens naturally, causing greater thinning and fragility of the vaginal walls. The vagina is not an open tunnel, I discovered. When you're grocery shopping or at a baseball game or otherwise not sexually aroused, your vagina is just a collapsed space. As you become excited, it gets longer and wider, like a balloon filling with air, and "sweats" the droplets of fluid that facilitate intercourse. But when your ovaries are removed and you're not producing estrogen, that swelling and lubrication take place more slowly, and sex can feel dry and uncomfortable, no matter how beloved, skilled, and considerate your partner.

Estrogen works its magic in the arousal phase, providing the lubrication that makes sex pleasurable rather than painful. But sexual *desire* in women is actually regulated by a weak form of the male hormone testosterone that is also made in the ovaries, and in the adrenal glands. After a hysterectomy, the adrenals may not keep up the production. Helen Singer Kaplan, a psychiatrist and director of the human sexuality program at New York Hospital–Cornell Medical Center in New York City, was a pioneer in testing to see whether a cancer patient who complains about loss of sexual interest is actually low in testosterone, a possibility that was virtually ignored by most doctors until recently. "The male medical establishment hates the idea of testosterone for women," she said in an article in *Bazaar* shortly before her death from breast cancer in 1996. "They act like it's putting a penis on women." But there's a sex center in the brain, just as there is an eating center and a sleep center, and it needs testosterone. Women need exactly 10 percent of what men need. With 10 percent, our sex centers are lively but we don't grow beards. Without it, a woman loses her libido, regardless how motivated she is psychologically.

Libido is not a high-priority issue to most doctors after diagnosing cancer. "Oncologists and gynecologists don't talk a lot about sexuality," says Allen Levine, a social worker and the assistant director of social services at Cancer Care, a counseling agency in New York City. "Physicians are concerned with saving lives, not with 'Are you getting any lately?'" In the hospital I was given a booklet called "Sexuality & Cancer" published by the American Cancer Society, a regular little *Joy of Sex* for the erotically challenged, complete with drawings of suggested positions and a blueprint for a "desire diary," in which to record when and where you have a sexual thought and what you did about it.

What I did was to call my gynecologist, who reaffirmed her place on my "best" list with her constructive strategy for my problem. I now take an estrogen-testosterone supplement called Estratest made by Solvay Pharmaceuticals in Marietta, Georgia. Technically, the drug is still awaiting FDA approval. When the FDA asked for proof that such a combination is effective, there was no proven method of measuring synthetic testosterone in the blood. New methods were developed and the data submitted to the FDA, but the drug remains in a kind of limbo—legally marketed, pronounced safe and effective by the manufacturer, but awaiting a stamp of approval from the nation's drug watchdog. I'd fight to the death before I'd let anyone take it out of my medicine cabinet. I'd always enjoyed a wonderful sex life, and it was dispiriting to have it evaporate. The hormone replacements made things . . . not perfect but okay, and I was assured by Carolyn Runowicz that there would be even more improvement as the specter of cancer faded. "It's the last horizon, the last thing you get back," she says. "It's not good enough just to have sex. You want passion. That comes from emotional healing."

I never talked about these personal issues with other cancer survivors. I probably alienated some perfectly nice people by firmly refusing all offers of support groups, and Andrew regularly turned down invitations to partake of "spousal support." I applaud the efforts of cancer veterans and their families who want to help one another, but I take no comfort in numbers. My husband is my support, and I am his. Perhaps our congenitally British stiff upper lips preclude accepting solace from strangers. Perhaps we thought of such unburdening as counterproductive wallowing, when we really wanted to move on. Perhaps the unique symbiosis of our long relationship doesn't allow another person to assume such an important role. I know the prevailing theory is that no one who has not been through it can truly understand this experience, but I felt so supported by my (mostly female) magazine staff. True, none of them had been through ovarian cancer, but they're *girls*, and they empathized in the most compassionate and unexpected ways. During my four months of chemo, from January to May, I always felt I was being heard and validated, no matter how bad things got.

In May 1994, Peter Dottino took forty-nine biopsies in a second-look procedure, determinedly searching like Hercule Poirot for any tiny malignant holdouts in my body. The aftermath was excru-ciating—I was bruised for many months afterward—but I was

31

declared cancer-free. Cancer treatment has become so much a work-in-progress that the "second-look surgery," which used to be a routine follow-up, has become controversial: Doctors don't have a lot to offer if the disease has returned, and it's still surgery, with all the attendant risks and assaults on the body: anesthesia, infections, swelling, pain. Most research concurs that the second look does not reduce the chance of recurrence or increase long-term survival. Such operations are now performed only as part of clinical trials, no longer standard care for ovarian cancer patients. Since I was included in such a trial, I had to consider what I would do with the information from the second look and decided that if more cancer was discovered, I would accept whatever further treatment was necessary.

From time to time now, I'll hear a female friend or colleague grouse about an upcoming gynecologist appointment, just as I used to do, and I realize how much I long for the days when such a checkup was inconvenient but prosaic, when the earth was still terra firma. I've rewritten history: Now "B.C." means "before cancer." I still go to the gynecologist—a lot of me is missing in action, but I do have breasts that need to be checked—and one day I noticed that she always pulled my chart from a small stack of manila folders on a shelf behind her desk, not the big file cabinets in the front office. The stack constitutes a private club: It's the records of all her patients with cancer, those who are still alive.

# 3

WE BEGIN HERE *ab ovo*, "from the egg," from the beginning. The narrative of ovarian cancer starts quite literally with the egg. The disease is thought to be a result of ovulation gone awry. In every woman, every month from menarche to menopause, one egg enlarges and ruptures near the surface of the ovary, where it awaits its fate: It may be fertilized by a congenial sperm and settle into the wall of the uterus on its way to becoming a baby, or it may be sloughed off as part of a period. Some women can feel when this happens, with a mid-cycle pang called *mittelschmerz*—I sometimes thought I felt it myself, a faint drumbeat of pain. But every time the egg blows through the ovary, the cells lining the surface have to divide and proliferate to fill in the hole left behind. It is in the normal, orderly repair of that hole (called, with some augury, a stigma) that cells can run amok and cancerous changes begin.

The statistics on ovarian cancer in the United States reveal a steady rise, gaining in momentum slowly but significantly over recent years, up to 1 in 55 women for 1997. (Earlier statistics are elusive because a misplaced sense of shame about "female problems" meant that the disease was often described as "stomach cancer.") And yet we're reminded by the experts that it's still relatively "rare," particularly for women under forty. (Dramatizing it for a character on the TV series *thirtysomething* was a statistical oddity, although this is cold comfort to the young women who are diagnosed with the disease.) Compare that 1 in 55 (which translates to a lifetime risk of 1.8 percent) to the figures for breast cancer (the widely quoted 1 in 8, or a lifetime risk of 12.5 percent), and it doesn't sound so menacing. But ovarian cancer is much, much deadlier, fatal in 60 percent of cases because three-quarters of the women diagnosed already have advanced disease. Ovarian cancer is classically described as a silent killer. The ovaries sit in a rather commodious abdominal cavity that can accommodate a lot of disease, undetected for too long. The symptoms are subtle and, because this cancer hits so many women in midlife, too often dismissed as a natural part of the aging process. The telltale tummy bulge is attributed to middle-age spread, the indigestion is blamed on spicy food, and the feeling of being full after a small meal is ascribed to a sluggish appetite. It seldom causes bleeding in postmenopausal women or changes the periods of younger menstruating women.

Several years ago the International Federation of Gynecology and Obstetrics established guidelines to determine the stage of disease and the recommended treatment: In Stage I, cancer is confined to one or both ovaries. In Stage II, it has spread to the uterus, fallopian tubes, or other tissues in the pelvis. (Stage II is actually quite rare because it would be unusual for cancer cells to detach from the ovaries but not travel past the belly button.) In Stage III, cancer is found in the lymph nodes of the abdomen or on the surface of other abdominal organs such as the liver, colon, or intestines. In Stage IV, it has penetrated those organs or spread beyond the abdominal area.

When ovarian cancer is detected early, the cure rate is high: at least a 90 percent five-year survival for Stage I diagnosis. At Stage IV, they tell you to go home and get your affairs in order.

Unlike the mammogram for breast cancer and the Pap smear

for cervical cancer, there is no routine ovarian cancer screening technique recommended and endorsed for widespread use. Even if you are a health-conscious person—if you take vitamins, get flu shots, floss daily, and have your various orifices poked and probed in regular checkups—you have little ammunition against ovarian cancer. It defies detection during a routine pelvic exam because what feels normal to the most experienced hands is so subjective.

Most women who contract ovarian cancer are postmenopausal. Since the ovaries tend to shrink after menopause, it has been suggested that a palpable ovary in a postmenopausal woman is in itself an alarm bell. But hands-on diagnosis depends on the average doctor's capacity to discriminate between an almond and a pecan simply by feel: A healthy ovary is about the size of an almond. If cancer is present, it's the size of a pecan, but by then there are already a *billion* cancer cells. The situation is complicated when a woman is, as I was, more queen-size than sylph. One of my doctors explained it this way: Think about placing a pecan on a mattress, then covering it with sheets and a thin blanket. If you run your hand over the top, it is probable that you would feel the pecan. Now put on a quilt and a bedspread, and think about the probability of feeling the pecan. Throw a grapefruit under there and you'll feel it, but by the time things are grapefruit-size, you're way into the danger zone. It's obvious why early detection would save lives, but there are only two imperfect and contentious possibilities for accomplishing that.

First there's the blood test that measures CA-125 antigens— those proteins shed by the cancer cells that induce an immune response. The test certainly has value: 80 percent of women with ovarian cancer will have an elevated CA-125 level, as I did. But one's CA-125 level can be raised by many benign conditions: menstruation, pregnancy, fibroids, cysts, endometriosis, pelvic inflammatory disease—anything that irritates the abdominal cavity. *Men* can have an elevated CA-125, and we know they don't have ovarian cancer. Because of the many false positives, the test is considered an inefficient tool for screening and diagnosis, with a huge potential to send a woman off on a merry-go-round of further evaluation that could end in invasive and perhaps unnecessary surgery. Once you have an elevated CA-125, there's no way of knowing whether the cause is ovarian cancer unless you have a laparoscopy, in which a thin telescopic tube is inserted to explore the pelvis. Even if the doctor doesn't detect cancer, you're left with the anxiety of an elevated CA-125 with no known cause. How far do you pursue it? What's your doctor's index of suspicion in taking care of you? Experts admit it's a tough, multifaceted problem. The only way to ascertain that you *don't* have ovarian cancer is to take out the ovaries, which in younger women means instant menopause.

The CA-125 test *is* useful in monitoring women who have already been treated for ovarian cancer, since a rising number can signal a recurrence of the disease. But the CA-125 level will be normal in more than half the women with Stage I disease, and in 20 percent of women at all other stages. The cancer may be composed of different kinds of cells, and some of them make what's detected by the CA-125 test, but some of them don't. Even the doctor whose laboratory developed the CA-125 test admits that it's not an appropriate one for screening the general population. "The call for widespread CA-125 testing is well intentioned but probably not the way to go," says Dr. Robert C. Bast, Jr., who heads the division of medicine at the University of Texas M. D. Anderson Cancer Center.

Two new blood tests, OVX-1 and MCFS, that are meant to be used in conjunction with a newer version of CA-125 have been developed by Bast's former colleagues at Duke University's Comprehensive Cancer Center in Durham, North Carolina. (OVX-1 is an antigen similar to CA-125, and MCFS is a growth factor secreted by some cancer cells.) Neither test is ready for the public, although the combination is promising.

Which leads us to the other screening tool: transvaginal sonography. One of the first things that happens to a woman with ovarian cancer is that her body forms new blood vessels. "Tumors are like little parasites," explains Dr. Beth Karlan, director of the Gilda Radner Ovarian Cancer Detection Program at the UCLA

School of Medicine. "They like to eat and need blood vessels to feed them. Tumor-associated blood vessels have different characteristics—they're like sump pumps." The sonogram uses a probe and color Doppler radar (like the weather report on the six o'clock news) to identify those vessels, along with volume and tissue patterns in the ovaries that appear abnormal. It's extremely reliable . in identifying a mass, but it cannot distinguish between benign and malignant, so it may lead down that same inevitable path to surgery.

The Gilda Radner detection program at UCLA honors the talented comedienne who died in 1989, at age forty-two, of ovarian cancer. Because of the value our society places on celebrity, it sometimes takes fame to focus attention on a health crisis, even posthumously—Rock Hudson did it for AIDS, John Belushi for drug addiction. Radner was one of less than 5 percent of women with a family history of the disease. One close relative with ovarian cancer means that your lifetime risk goes from 1.8 to 5 percent; two relatives takes it to 7 percent. (It's important to know about your father's side of the family as well: The genetic mutation that may lead to cancer can be inherited from either parent.) Scientists have recently been able to identify more than a hundred possible mutations of a gene called BRCA-1 that carries a 40 to 60 percent risk of ovarian cancer and an 80 to 85 percent risk of breast cancer. Another gene, called BRCA-2, also confers an 80 percent risk of breast cancer and a 20 percent risk of ovarian cancer. When these high-risk women do *not* develop cancer, it is thought that there may be other protective genes blocking the malignant growth.

ALL OF US have cancer cells in our bodies that our immune system routinely ferrets out and destroys, according to Dr. Adriane Fugh-Berman, chairman of the National Women's Health Network in Washington, D.C. It is likely to be the interaction between cancer cells and your immune system that determines your medical fate. Women who develop ovarian cancer despite having no family history of the disease may be the victims of bad luck, but there's

37

bad and then there's worse. The overwhelming majority of ovarian cancers are deemed "sporadic," meaning there is no evidence of genetic susceptibility. Our own habits and decisions may be implicated in our fortunes.

Ovarian cancer has been linked to a typical Western high-fat diet, like the red meat, fried eggs, and buttered sandwiches (on sliced white bread—like Mother's Pride, the English version of Wonder Bread that I grew up on in Britain). The lowest incidence of the disease is in Japan, Hong Kong, and Singapore, but when Asian women emigrate here and start substituting cheeseburgers for sushi, they move right up in the statistics. In 1984, the Harvard Medical School conducted a study comparing the fat, alcohol, coffee, and smoking profiles of women with ovarian cancer and a similar group of healthy women. The only significant difference was that the women with ovarian cancer were more likely to use whole milk and butter. A 1994 study from Yale University found that the risk of ovarian cancer goes up 20 percent for every 10 grams of saturated fat consumed daily, and 42 percent for every 100 milligrams of egg cholesterol (one large egg has about 212 milligrams of cholesterol). But the risk goes down by 37 percent for every 10 grams of vegetable fiber consumed. (Fruit fiber doesn't seem to convey this benefit.)

Ovarian cancer is most common in countries with the highest consumption of dairy products, particularly cottage cheese and yogurt, which contain a sugar called galactose that is already broken down and doesn't even have to be digested by the body. Women who are dairy-intolerant, as many Asians are, are at lower risk. When galactose is fed to female laboratory rats, their ovaries shrink and their eggs die, and if the rat is pregnant, the galactose kills the eggs of her unborn daughter.

There is a relatively low rate of ovarian cancer in Mediterranean countries, which some researchers attribute to their copious use of olive oil. A 1993 study from Greece compared the dietary habits of about 200 hospitalized ovarian cancer patients to an equal number of healthy women just visiting the hospitals and found that olive oil (the amounts are not clear) lowered the risk by approximately 20 percent.

Of course, cheeseburgers and milkshakes are manifestly, nakedly wicked, and one could hardly be surprised that they're not health promoters. But some risk factors are more insidious. Who would have dreamed that baby powder could be hazardous? It turns out that talc is chemically similar to asbestos, a known carcinogen (both are magnesium silicates), and some cosmetic talc is contaminated by asbestos from nearby mines. Powder that is dusted on underwear, sanitary napkins, or diaphragms could travel through the vagina and cervix into the uterus and through the fallopian tubes to the ovaries. In 1976, manufacturers voluntarily limited the amount of asbestos permitted in talcum power (so nice of them), but it's still used on most condoms produced in this and other countries, which means repeated exposure for some women. Studies continue to show an association between ovarian cancer and talc long past the time when asbestos should be a concern, indicating that the talc itself may induce a foreign-body response. Three recent studies from Harvard, Yale, and the Fred Hutchinson Cancer Research Center in Seattle concluded that a lifetime pattern of using talc near the genital area, including the ever-popular "feminine hygiene sprays," may increase the risk of ovarian cancer. The FDA is still evaluating this research.

Emotions may be inculpated in ovarian cancer as in other diseases. The mind–body connection is now widely accepted in medicine, even among the most conservative of scientists. We blush with embarrassment, get headaches from tension, and doctors recognize the healing powers of the placebo: a counterfeit, impotent pill that nevertheless generates a "cure" in an astonishing number of people who think it is medicine. I'm certainly willing to believe that, to fracture an old song lyric, the head bone's connected to the hip bone. I've heard the theory that ovarian cancer may result from the energy of unexpressed rage or resentment, emanating from the "second chakra" of the body, and I've seen some good science suggesting that depressed or repressed people are more likely to develop any kind of cancer. One study at the renowned Johns Hopkins Medical Center in Baltimore found that cancer patients were more detached from their parents, had more negative attitudes about their families, and tended to bottle up their emotions.

WHILE ALL OF these studies provide interesting expository tidbits, it's unlikely that something like yogurt or anger will prove to be statistically significant in the development of ovarian cancer; otherwise, the disease would be much, much more prevalent. The studies go on, but whatever your mental health, eating habits, hygiene or contraceptive practices, the one consistent risk factor for ovarian cancer for *every* woman seems to be ovulation. The more often ovaries go through the stress of a monthly cycle that ends in the rupture of an egg, the more prone they are to damage, and to the development of abnormal cells that can become cancer. One of the lowest rates of ovarian cancer is in women with Turner's syndrome, a genetic abnormality in women whereby an X-chromosome is missing, so they're sterile and don't ovulate. On the other hand, *chickens*, which ovulate all the time—they make an egg every day—have a *high* rate of ovarian cancer.

Anything that suppresses ovulation temporarily confers some protection: Pregnancy, breast-feeding, and oral contraceptives all give your ovaries time off. When you're pregnant, the high level of hormones in the placenta shuts down normal ovarian function. Studies have found that each child decreases your risk of ovarian cancer by 14 percent. A study done by the Centers for Disease Control in Atlanta showed that the longer a woman used birth-control pills, which simulate the hormones of pregnancy, the lower her risk of ovarian cancer. The CDC estimated that more than 1,700 cases in the United States are averted each year by the Pill. (The Pill, however, carries with it certain risks, the most serious of which is the chance of cardiovascular disease for certain groups of women older than thirty-five, obese women, those with high blood pressure or high cholesterol, and smokers.)

But what about the reverse? If ovarian cancer is associated with what is called "incessant ovulation," it would seem to make sense that the *hyperovulation* caused by fertility drugs means a higher risk. A few reports trickled into the medical literature of the 1980s about women who developed ovarian cancer after being treated for infertility. But it's only in recent years that enough women have taken these drugs to make epidemiologic studies possible. In 1992, pooling data from three previous studies, Dr. Alice Whittemore at Stanford University found that women who had been treated for infertility and went on to have children were 3 times more likely to develop ovarian cancer, and women who were treated but never became pregnant were at 27 times greater risk.

When Whittemore's work was published, all hell broke loose in the fertility community. Women desperate to have a baby were panicked, and the specialists who treated them were horrified that they might be endangering their patients, not to mention their lucrative business. Whittemore was attacked as the anti–Christ and her research labeled well-meaning sophistry. Whittemore herself considers the study inconclusive. Since non-motherhood, whether by choice or chance, puts women at more risk for ovarian cancer, it's not clear whether the study was documenting risk for the can't-get-pregnant or simply the never-been-pregnant. It's possible the infertile women had a defect of the ovaries that not only prevented them from getting pregnant but also brought about the malignancy. *And* the study simply reflected women who could not get pregnant for any reason, not filtering out what are called "male factors"— in other words, women with blocked fallopian tubes were clumped together with women whose husbands had low sperm counts.

The Whittemore study was never designed to look for a risk from fertility drugs. "We had a huge sample of women with ovarian cancer and a comparable sample without ovarian cancer," she says, "and we asked them a whole battery of questions trying to get at what may be causing the disease. Fertility treatment was only one small part." Most of the women interviewed were over sixty, so they'd been trying to get pregnant during a time when infertility was treated with anything from steroids to thyroid medication to radiation to DES (diethylstilbestrol), the synthetic hormone later implicated in severe birth defects. (Clomid and Pergonal, the drugs that I took and that are in common use today, were not approved and on the market in a big way until much later. Clomid was approved in the U.S. in 1967, in the U.K. in 1972. Pergonal was approved first in the U.K. in 1969, in the U.S. in 1975.) But the study did not differentiate between the various treatments in common use at that time, nor did it indicate whether the women had been treated for weeks or months or years. Some of the women couldn't even remember what they'd been given—they just knew they took *something*.

Whittemore points out another major problem in trying to find a link between ovarian cancer and infertility treatment from her study: A lot of these women were very, very ill with ovarian cancer. And when you've got a life-threatening disease, you may remember things differently than if you were interviewed between tennis sets. In science, that's known as a recall bias. What was needed was research that did not depend on memory but on fact, taken from medical records.

Enter Dr. Mary Anne Rossing, an epidemiologist at the Fred Hutchinson Cancer Research Center. Rossing studied 4,000 American women who were treated for infertility in the 1970s and 1980s. Among those women who had taken Clomid for 12 or more cycles (which would mean at least one year), the relative risk of developing ovarian cancer was increased 11 times. (Since Clomid was approved in the U.S. before Pergonal, it was the only drug in sufficient use to evaluate.) Despite causing this further shakeup of the fertility community, Rossing was not subjected to the kind of vitriol that had been directed at Whittemore by the specialists routinely prescribing the drugs. "They'd had a chance to lose their emotions about it," she says, "and maybe realized it was an issue that deserved further study." Which is exactly what Rossing is doing in two ongoing studies funded by the National Institute of Child Health and Human Development. One will involve about 2,500 women in Seattle, Detroit, and Atlanta, comparing previous use of fertility drugs by healthy women and by those with ovarian cancer. Information about the types, dosage, and duration of treatment will be taken directly from the records of fertility clinics, and blood samples will be taken from the participants to test for the BRCA-1 gene. The other study will look at the incidence of ovarian cancer in 12,000 women in the Seattle area, all of whom were diagnosed as infertile, to determine whether more women in the group that went on to treatment developed cancer. (If the treatment carries no more risk than does the fact of infertility itself, you would expect to see no difference between the two groups of women.)

It turns out that Gilda Radner took fertility drugs too. Her husband, the actor Gene Wilder, who'd served in the Army Medical Corps, gave her shots of Pergonal himself, after practicing first on oranges and grapefruits.


TO GRASP THE potentially awesome effect of fertility drugs, it's necessary to go back to what the ovaries do. Perhaps you'll be as surprised as I was to learn that a woman is actually born with all the eggs she'll ever have. The egg count is several million as a fetus, dwindling to about 400,000 by the time you begin to menstruate, and they die off at the rate of about 1,000 a month through a natural, perfectly normal process of age-related cellular death called atresia.

Every month from the time of puberty, the hypothalamus, a thumb-size gland at the base of the brain, secretes a chemical messenger called GnRH (gonadotropin-releasing hormone), which signals the neighboring pituitary gland (about the size of a fingertip) to make two hormones: FSH (follicle-stimulating hormone) encourages the development of a dominant follicle (occasionally two, ergo twins) in one of the ovaries, and LH (luteinizing hormone) causes that follicle to release an egg (ovulation). Another hormone called inhibin is produced in the developing follicles in response to FSH: The one with the most inhibin "inhibits" the other follicles and becomes the champ. The released egg is picked up by the fingerlike projections called fimbria on the nearest fallopian tube, where it may be fertilized by a friendly sperm that happens to be in the neighborhood, and the fimbria act as a sort of benevolent crossing guard in waving the egg along to the uterus. The maturing follicle, now called a corpus luteum (Latin for "yellowish body," because of its color), makes estrogen, which builds up the endometrium (lining of the uterus) in case it's needed to nourish an embryo, and progesterone, which stabilizes that thickened tissue. If the corpus luteum isn't fertilized, it dies like so many other eggs, and without the supply of hormones the uterine lining collapses, to be shed as a menstrual period.

But suppose this intricate and elegant system breaks down? Modern science has provided a means of intervention: ovulation induction. Clomid is an *anti-estrogen*. It sends a false message to the brain, tricking it into thinking there's less estrogen around than there really is, so the pituitary goes into overdrive producing FSH, urging the follicles in the ovaries to develop and start making estrogen. With all that stimulation, more eggs are likely to be released. Pergonal acts somewhat differently, by *substituting* for FSH and LH to stimulate the ovaries into producing several mature eggs, rather than waiting for the pituitary to make these hormones on its own. Known in medicalese as hMG, or human menopausal gonadotropins, it used to be extracted from the urine of post-menopausal nuns in Italy (I'm not kidding), but now it can be manufactured. Either drug may be boosted by injections of a hormone called hCG (human chorionic gonadotropin), which is secreted by the placenta in early pregnancy and mimics the pituitary's own LH. (When you take a pregnancy test, either in your doctor's office or in your own bathroom with a kit, what's being measured is your hCG level.)

There are other fertility drugs, abstrusely named and less frequently prescribed—I've just detailed the superstars. With these modern medicines, it is possible to usurp the prerogative of God or Mother Nature or whoever you like to believe is responsible for these things, blasting the ovaries and playing jokes on the brain.

I had this done nine times.

# 4

POPULAR PSYCHOLOGY HOLDS that the most potent weapon
against cancer is a "positive attitude," but it can't be turned on at
will. Real second-nature optimism comes, I think, directly from
upbringing, and I had the best possible start in life. I grew up in
three of Britain's most beautiful counties: first Herefordshire on
the border of Wales, with big-horned Jacob sheep grazing on the
Black Mountains in the distance; then Bath in Somerset, with its
golden-mellow classical architecture by John D. Wood the Elder;
and boarding school in Worcestershire, the apple-growing part of
England, with dappled orchards and rolling green hills. I was a
boisterous, well-adjusted girl who put down roots at school without
a twinge of trauma. It could so easily have been the kind of safe,
unimaginative upbringing shared by so many girls of my class and
generation, leading to comfy, stolid marriage and motherhood.
But my family has an odd and original streak that gave me experiences and values way beyond the grasp of most British children of
the 1950s and 1960s.

I was born September 7, 1947, in my maternal grandfather's

rambling nineteenth-century house in Alderley Edge, a posh village outside Manchester in the northwest corner of England. It was renowned for its coven of witches, who were rumored to gather near the cliffs on moonlit nights. My mother wanted to get out of the house that Indian summer's day to see a new show at the theater in Manchester, but the midwife forbade her to travel, so instead of seeing *Oklahoma!* she had me. The moment I arrived, my grandfather charged onto the lawn and ran a flag up the pole—the Scottish flag. I imagine my mother sitting up in bed, holding her firstborn in a room perfumed with gladioli, my father, full of pride but furious about that damned flag, standing at her side.

My father, an ophthalmologist named Thomas Stuart-Black Kelly, considered himself to be Manx, a native of the Isle of Man, a small island in the Irish Sea between Scotland and Ireland with its own government and its own flag, perhaps the weirdest one ever unfurled: three running legs joined in the center, symbolizing a pre-Christian legend about a three-legged man who lived under a waterfall. Manx people aren't Scottish or English, and they aren't Welsh, and they most certainly are not Irish—my father hated when our surname was confused with the Irish Kellys. What they are is ancient Celt with a strong dash of Viking invader. That provenance explains a lot about my dear father: He was as hot-headed as a marauding Norseman when it came to expressing his idiosyncratic ideas, but had the welcoming and open-hearted Celtic spirit. We loved each other madly but fought like cats and dogs. During my teenage years, our rows were so explosive that my mother could scarcely guess which one of us would be alive when she got home. At mealtimes, my father would lead "P.C."—polite conversation. The subject could be starvation in Africa or black holes in space or the latest surgical bandaging techniques, but he'd never take a lazy, un-thought-out argument from any of us. "Always question what people tell you!" he'd shout. "You can say no to the system! It may have been the system for three hundred years, but that doesn't make it right."

For all my father's bombast, he had an extraordinary ability to charm and motivate everyone who worked for him; he was always scrupulous in showing courtesy and never patronizing. Formal "good manners" are taught to British children, but often they're meant to deflect real involvement, with graciousness substituting for intimacy. My father got involved with everybody, and watching him, I learned about artful solicitude and empathy. He had a talent for seeing where people came from in life, what their difficulties might be and how to encourage the best in them. Since I've been living in the United States, I've come to realize that the respect for people my father drilled into me is much more American than British. It has always stood me in good stead. When I was still a junior assistant underling at British *Vogue*, scurrying around photography studios tending to the well-being of everyone from the van driver to the hairdresser's assistant, my superiors would watch with astonishment. My breezy egalitarian manner was not at all normal for young ladies of my background. The distinguished "gentleman photographer" Norman Parkinson once took me aside and said, "You know, Liz, you're so good with the little people."

But my father was a paradox, espousing a number of reactionary ideas against which I argued and rebelled vociferously. He believed in racial separatism, a concept he patently contradicted by being a kind and generous employer of many black hospital workers. The scope of my father's intractable racial animus was broad enough to take in Greeks, and I chose to marry one: Andrew's parents are Greek Cypriots who met after their families moved to Britain in the 1930s. The day my father categorically forbade me to marry Andrew, I chucked the Minton china at him. It wasn't a good moment in our relationship, but I got my way. "There's only a bit of Manx in Elizabeth," my mother would say, "but it makes an awful lot of noise."

My mother's family were the Caldwells, who had made their money in the dyeing industry in Paisley, Scotland, the town that lent its name to the swirling patterns of abstract curves. Eventually my grandfather moved close to Manchester, the garment center of England, and became the managing director of the British Cotton and Wool Dyers Association. My mother Janet, her elder sister, and her younger brother were brought up in patrician affluence.

47

Alderley Edge was a picturesque village that began to attract wealthy industrialists at the turn of the century, and it still does: The area was recently noted as having the highest density of millionaires in Britain and the biggest per capita consumption of champagne. I suppose the nearest American comparison would be a sort of Victorian Beverly Hills. When my mother was a girl, the Caldwells had upstairs and downstairs maids, a cook and a chauffeur. Their house, called Meadscroft, had an orchid greenhouse on a manicured lawn and trellises of roses leading down to a pond where, as a child, I skipped about with my girl cousins in fairy wings made of green silk tulle and opalescent sequins.

When my grandfather died in the 1960s, the property was sold off and three new houses were built on the front lot. With my mother's inheritance and my father's income as an eye surgeon, our family was comfortably well-off, but the resources were rapidly eaten up by school and college tuition fees for me, my brother, Grant, and my sister, Lois. By the time I went off to British *Vogue*, I knew I had to live on what I earned. I had the right sort of background but none of the private income taken for granted by the other young women there, who accepted their pittance of a salary for the sheer joy and glamour of standing around the coffee machine. (There was a joke about an assistant who announced one day, "I have to get a real job. Daddy can't afford to send me to *Vogue* anymore.") And a need for thrift at that stage of life was not at all detrimental for me. The effort required to earn a living was motivation to accomplish what I might otherwise never have achieved.

I wonder if the Caldwell genes predisposed me to fashion. I inherited my aunt's childhood passion for making doll clothes, and my mother spent freely on her wardrobe before the constraints of putting three children through school made her more budget-conscious. I was intoxicated by the romance of her Horrocks' floral print dresses, Harris tweed suits, felt Trilby hats (a new one every time she went to a wedding), and her perfume, Je Reviens by Jean Patou. My parents had a rather glitzy social life, going to formal parties on rural estates and driving home by the light of the stars, so my mother owned lots of extravagant evening gowns—one in green grosgrain taffeta with pink and yellow embossing and flocking, one in black chantilly lace over midnight satin, and a red balloon dress caught under the knee, a radical shape for the time. It was all inspired by Christian Dior, whose pervasive influence reached even the far-flung provinces of England in the 1950s, and redefined the way women everywhere wanted to dress.

The appeal of all those gorgeous, feminine, swirly clothes for women like my mother must have been enormous after the war. My parents had met at a dance and married in 1940, and my father was conscripted into the army the next year, serving in the Far East. My mother spent the war years in the uniform of the Women's Army Transport Corps, where she became a fully trained mechanic and shuttled colonels in American Dodge trucks while the bombs fell, often at night. It was dangerous stuff, but she loved driving and navigating in unknown territory. In another life, she'd have liked to pursue her talent for map-reading and become a cartographer, but career expectations for married servicewomen came to an abrupt end when the war was over. Daddy was away for so long that Mummy worried whether she'd recognize the man she was going to meet at Paddington Station when he was finally sent home. In fact, my father *had* changed. He was the son of a Methodist lay preacher, brought up with strict religious beliefs, but he could never believe in a God of love after what he'd seen in the war. (One of his friends, who was also my godfather, was more severely damaged by those years: He had served with the "Dam Busters," the RAF planes that bombed the German power plants in the Ruhr Valley, and he was so haunted by the experience that he would periodically get roaring drunk, go out to the garden, and eat flowers. He preferred daffodils.)

I was born the year after my father came home, and the family moved to Shirehampton, on the outskirts of Bristol, where my father worked at the Royal Eye Infirmary and we lived in a little white house on the village green. One of my earliest memories, which has passed into family folklore, is of dragging a blanket off my bed and wearing it like a cape, positioned at the top of the stairs with my face pressed between the banisters, dying to join the party in the parlor. "Mummy," I would plead, "blanket-round-downstairs!" Even before I could talk properly, I couldn't stand being left out, and to this day I have a horror of being excluded or feeling alone—I like to be at the center of activity, surrounded by friends. Perhaps it was something else I got from Daddy: Our house was full of people because he'd been a lonely only child.

When I was three, my brother, Grant, was born, and we moved to Hereford, one of the place names Eliza Doolittle had to pronounce for her elocution lessons with Henry Higgins ("In Hartford, Hereford, and Hampshire, hurricanes hardly happen"). We had a red brick house called Penn-y-Bryn, which means "top of the hill" in Welsh, with a tiered garden ending in a row of tall poplars and a grassy lawn set up for tennis. My mother made crabapple tarts with fruit from a tree whose branches bent to touch the ground and told us stories about a hen named Clara Clutterbuck, and we played duets on the piano, "Autumn Leaves" and "March of the Queen of Sheba." I always loved dressing up—I was painting my lips with red Smarties candies at age five—and my father built me a white hardboard playhouse (called a "Wendy house," from *Peter Pan*). I was the impresario for a peewee theater troupe in our thatched-roof summerhouse—we'd rehearse all day, charge our parents admission, and sell lemonade at intermission. But we were forbidden to play on Sundays: In another of my father's peculiar mixed messages, he had virtually abandoned religion but observed the day of rest.

Only one family down the road had television, and we joined them to watch the coronation of Queen Elizabeth II in 1953—the same year my sister, Lois, was born. I was too young to be saddened by the recent death of King George VI, but I was mesmerized by the pretty young queen's dress, embroidered with the white rose of Yorkshire, the pink rose of Lancashire, the daffodil from Wales, the Scottish thistle, the Irish shamrock. And I was thrilled with the coronation gift souvenir bought for me by my parents: a golden toy coach with soldiers in red coats and black hats on white horses.

But television was a rarity. For entertainment I was much more likely to climb on the roof and wave signal flags or make "fairy gardens," fashioning doll figures out of red poppies and weaving thrones out of long grasses and berries. There was a steep slope at the side of the house leading to a rose garden, and down that slope my friends and I would push Grant in a crate fitted with wheels, angling it so the poor child would end up in the rose bushes and chasing him until his diapers fell down. One friend of the family tried to teach Grant self-defense. "Why don't you just get a big stick," she'd say to him, "and chase them back?" When we wanted to escape disciplining, we'd hide in the huge pots used for growing rhubarb. There was a vast patch of raspberries too, covered with netting so the birds couldn't get them, and long beds of asparagus, and a woodshed with white clematis and tomato vines creeping up the walls.

The colors of that garden are so deeply etched on my memory that they triggered an epiphany when I was in my twenties. I was reminded of the time I'd picked daffodils for the visiting nurse who'd come to tend my mother when I was a little girl. But why was the nurse there in springtime? None of us was born in the spring. My mother had had a miscarriage, of course. Nothing was said at the time. Like everything else in those days, it was just ... handled. My mother had an awful time trying to have babies, but she never showed us sorrow or self-pity. "Do you know," she told me only recently, "when I had Lois, it was the eighth time I'd been pregnant?"

At five, I started school at the Margaret Allen Preparatory, known as The Redcaps for our winter uniforms of scarlet beanies worn with navy mackintoshes, but it was the summertime outfits I loved: Panama hats with red ribbons and red-and-white polka-dotted dresses with big bows at the back. I was such a *girl*. My mother made my non-uniform clothes, favoring puffed sleeves and dirndl skirts, according to the fashion of the times. With postwar rationing still in effect, all my store-bought clothes came in care packages from American friends and relatives (my favorite for years was a red party dress with a lace collar and white angora bolero).

Special foods, such as canned hams and powdered eggs, arrived in these packages too. By law, all children had their diet supplemented with foul-tasting cod liver oil, dispensed by a government nurse. There were pantries in our basement, with plots of mushrooms growing in the dark, apples and potatoes stored in straw, braces of pheasants and pigeons, and perhaps a hank of venison given to my father by a grateful patient. It was all the bounty of the land—we never had exotica like grapes or cherries until many years later, and a chicken was only Christmas fare. One day my mother saw a line forming outside a shop and waited for an hour to buy one lemon, an item so foreign that when it was placed on the plate, we greeted it with hoots of derision. Afternoon tea was beans on toast, served by a succession of maids who were Welsh gypsies and had to receive instruction on how to set a table. I was driven to and from school in my mother's old Austin, but on Wednesdays I was allowed to walk home from school with my friends, stopping at a sweetshop for my quintessential childhood treat: an ice cream cone with a chocolate Milk Flake bar dipped into it.

On spring vacations, a great gang of our endlessly extended family—aunts and uncles and dozens of cousins and pretend-cousins and dogs and cats—would travel in a convoy of motorboats around the Norfolk Broads, the marshy and mysterious waterways on the east coast of Britain. We'd set off in the morning, decide where to meet up for supper, and play cards in the evening—not too exciting, except when one of the dogs tried to step from boat to shore, hind legs on the dinghy, front legs on the bank, getting longer and longer until she fell into the water. Sometimes we'd visit my grandparents on the Isle of Man, driving to Liverpool and through the Mersey Tunnel (we felt a deep kinship with Gerry and the Pacemakers when they recorded "Ferry 'Cross the Mersey"), then onto the wood-paneled Manx Steampacket Ferry, with a lunch of fish and chips served on white tablecloths. We'd drive the car off on the other side and proceed to the town of Peel, with its lugubrious medieval castle built to keep the Irish out. The ghost of Peel Castle is a large black dog, seen especially by people returning from the pub, and the beautiful waterfalls nearby are

home to leprechauns. Early in life I memorized William Alling-
ham's poem "The Fairies," which starts "Up the airy mountain, /
Down the rushy glen, / We daren't go a-hunting / For fear of little
men." Sometimes we'd visit the Gower Peninsula in South Wales,
where we'd stay in boardinghouses and eat seaweed for breakfast.
Once we rented an old railway carriage that had been turned into
a vacation home. It was one of those idyllic, gentle childhoods,
and maybe they still exist in Britain, but I doubt it. It was safe. It
was always sunny. There was no pressure outside of school. And
nothing ever seemed to happen.

In my last year at The Redcaps, Daddy got a serious travel bug.
Like all Manxmen, who've been setting out from their tiny island
for centuries to explore and survive, he had an adventurous wan-
derlust. Ever resourceful and blessed with a surgeon's skilled hands,
he built an extraordinary family-size car by welding together half
of a bottle-green Jaguar convertible (bought secondhand for cheap)
and half of a station wagon. This splendid hybrid was quite roomy,
and our family of five could travel anywhere, starting with America.
The British middle class didn't stray far from home at that time;
and few people had ever been abroad: Only the wealthy could
afford plane fare, and package holidays were nonexistent. What
limited information people had about the outside world came from
cinema newsreels, newspapers, and magazines. I had no sense
that my experience was remarkable—or that my father's can-do
attitude, which I happened to inherit, was anything out of the
ordinary.

It was April 1957, I was nearly ten, Grant seven, and Lois four,
when we tackled the United States. I'd always thought that the
sole and serious purpose of this trip was for my father to exchange
information on retinal detachment with American eye surgeons
and academics, but recently I asked my mother why we'd gone to
America, and she said, "We went to look at it!" We drove our
green hybrid to Southampton and watched, scarcely breathing, as
the car was hoisted onto the Cunard Line's S.S. *Britannic.* The
Atlantic crossing was turbulent as we skirted hurricanes, and the
troughs between the waves were as big as the ship. But we managed

to have fun, even down in steerage, with sirens going off for lifeboat drills, and consommé served midmorning on deck, and movies shown every day after lunch. (I had seen only two movies in my life up till then, *Snow White* and *Sleeping Beauty*.) My brother took boxing lessons, and I swam in a frigid pool the size of a baptismal font, and everybody said how beautiful our teeth were. When we sailed into New York Harbor, we were watching the Statue of Liberty on one side of the ship, when my father scooped us up and said, "Come look at the other side." And there was Manhattan. Night was falling, as was a spring snow, and through the flurries we could see thousands of lights towering into the sky. By extraordinary coincidence, when I look out my office window today, I can see Pier 54 on the Hudson River, the exact spot where we landed forty years ago. And just across the street from my office is the Wellington Hotel (now the Ameritania), where we spent the first nights of our American adventure.

We made our way cross-country by looking for the oldest, shabbiest motels, we three children in sleeping bags on the floor, and staying with relatives where we could. Currency regulations allowed us to take only 100 pounds per adult and 70 pounds for each child—that was about $600 for six weeks, a situation that called for economy measures but was hardly a problem for a woman who'd been through wartime rationing as the bombs fell on Britain. My mother cooked up an unwavering diet of Spam, canned beans, and bacon on a camp stove in the motel rooms. "It was strictly forbidden, of course," she now says blithely. "And we all got a bit thin."

We fared better when we stayed with various Kellys who had struck out for America before us, beginning around the turn of the century. That side of the family produced a line of strong, smart, entrepreneurial women who flourished in a way that would never have been possible in England, let alone a tiny farming community on the Isle of Man. Great Aunt Isabel was an anthropologist who was living in Mexico and working for the U.S. government as a troubleshooter in foreign countries where the welfare of women was jeopardized. Because of her training, she understood the customs and traditions of places like Pakistan and Bolivia—the significance of color in their clothing, for example, or why they might be reluctant to accept Western medical care for themselves or their children. Great Aunt Eve owned a dress shop in Santa Cruz (naturally a much more compelling enterprise to me). Cousin Mona got started in business when, bored by house-wifery, she bought a cow, the brunt of her husband's jokes until she sold the animal for twice what she'd paid for it. After that, Mona just "branched out." She was the first person in California to raise polled Herefords (cows without horns are gentler beasts in a herd), becoming owner of her own ranch in Santa Rosa and later heading the Cowbelles, a female ranchers' association.

So we drove across America to see the cousins: from the historic landmarks of Philadelphia and Washington, D.C., through the Blue Ridge Mountains (where we got our first look at a skunk) to the Carolinas, across the Texas panhandle on Route 66, up through the Grand Canyon and Hoover Dam, visiting ghost towns with tumbleweed blowing through the streets, into the Petrified Forest and over the Painted Desert, where I got a glass tube filled with colored sands, on to Los Angeles and Disneyland, where I rode a rocket to "outer space." We sang "She'll Be Comin' 'Round the Mountain" and "Cumberland Gap" and "The Black Hills of Dakota" like Doris Day; we ate hot dogs and watched motel-room TV and gave puppet shows for each other in the back of the car. I was much more impressed by a huge suburban supermarket or a dead snake on the road than by the Liberty Bell or the White House. Happiness was stopping at a different coffee shop every day for our "elevenses" (midmorning snack) and the purchase one day of a new doll, a "Miss America Barbie," who had thick blond ponytails and large bosoms. When we got to Cousin Eve's house, I went to school with her daughter Susan, but I wouldn't say the Pledge of Allegiance, terrified that I'd be stripped of my British citizenship and denied passage home with my family. And I was bitterly disappointed that there were no cowboys or Indians at Cousin Mona's ranch, having read about the American Wild West and acted out those parts in our backyard plays. Prophetically, we even visited the Hearst castle at San Simeon, a glorious folly of Pompeian tiles and Flemish tapestries, gilded doorways and hand-carved choir stalls. My parents explained about Hearst as the putative inspiration for *Citizen Kane*, but I didn't know that one day the name would be on my paycheck.

We returned by way of the waterfalls at Yosemite and Yellow-stone National Park, where bears crawled all over the car. From there we went to Salt Lake City, where I was fascinated by the acoustics of the Mormon Tabernacle—a pin dropped at one end could be heard at the other—then across the Mississippi, which I was proud to spell correctly in the diary I was keeping. Also noted in the diary is the fact that "many of the people in Chicago are black," the last word crossed out and replaced with "Negroes"—an early attempt to be politically correct. We went under the Horseshoe Falls at Niagara and bought presents in New York City at "a big shop called Macy's," as the diarist recorded. Back home, I discovered that I was a celebrity at school. Traveling all over America at the age of ten was a singular experience, even by today's standards, and in 1950s England it was like going to the moon. When I told the story of our American odyssey to Claeys Bahrenburg, who hired me for *Harper's Bazaar*, he felt somewhat reassured about my transplantability from Britain to the States. If someone says, "It's not going to play in Nebraska," I know about that—*and* about that big shop called Macy's.

FROM THE FIRST moment I drew breath, there was never any doubt that at the age of eleven I would go to boarding school at Malvern Girls' College—my mother had been there in the 1920s, and that was that. Malvern is a genteel Victorian town that used to have a mineral spa, set in landscapes that inspired the lyrical musical compositions of Edward Elgar. The Girls' College, unfortunately known as the Ugly 500, was housed in an ivy-clad building that had once been a railway hotel, but the amenities were more along the lines of boot camp. There was no hot water in the dormitories, just jugs and basins from which to wash. We were allowed to take baths twice a week and do laundry once a week, which meant wearing our allotted five pairs of underpants (called knicker linings) more than once. Permission to leave school on a weekend, called an exeat, was issued only three times a term. At the sound of a gong, we filed into the dining hall for meals, forbidden to touch the polished oak banisters on the stairs, and we put our hands out for inspection by a prefect. Mail was distributed in a daily roll call at two o'clock—my memory is triggered whenever I see a similar scene in a film about prison life or the military.

It sounds rather grim and dour, but at the time it was an adventure and I loved it. So many generations of boys and girls have been permanently warped by the British public school system (it has always amused me that the American term "private school" and the English term "public school" mean exactly the same thing)—its rigid rules of conduct, its emphasis on ancient regimes, its insular order of caste and class, its *Prime of Miss Jean Brodie* undercurrents of repressed sexuality. But I liked the starchy food, the stews and breaded cutlets and the pastries called Chelsea buns that were rolled up with sugar and currants. (I once ate nine of those in fifteen minutes to win a contest.) I liked the teachers we called "Latin Willie" and "Miss Mucky Cow" (McCowan). I liked the assembly at the start of every day, with the entire school population reciting "Our Father who art in Heaven ...," and the compulsory services at the Priory on Sundays, when we wore felt skirts, pastel cotton shirts with striped ties that featured our house color (mine was orange), garter belts with 60-denier stockings and brogues. I learned to play the wind organ at the church next to the school. As a tone-deaf youngster, I took music lessons to improve my tin ear and actually turned out to have a gift for the piano. I liked the sound of fifty girls at piano practice in the tiny rooms of the music corridor under the eaves of the school, the evidence of their mediocre skills carrying out into quad and all the way to the railway station. I even liked the discipline, because I could fight it—it wasn't possible to be *really* bad, but I could be defiant.

At age twelve, I told Canon Lunt at the Malvern Abbey that I could not be confirmed because I didn't believe in God. When I went out to buy some confirmation cards for friends, I realized that I thought the whole process was silly. My insolence was reported to my father, who said, "If that's what she wants, that's all right," and the pastor must have washed his hands of the whole family. Certainly I had absorbed my father's agnosticism and spurned the notion of blind faith. I learned from him to believe what my eyes and ears reveal. I've always wanted to be part of things but also to preserve my individuality. That's still an important dichotomy that informs my decisions.

Malvern was known for academic excellence, for the alumnae who went on to become doctors, physicists, and the first female judge in Britain, but I was never a scholar. Year after year, my report cards always had the same lukewarm praise: "Elizabeth tries hard." I was not expected to follow my father into medicine—he had told me point-blank, "You will not be a doctor, because you will only get married and waste the education"—but art, my first love and natural talent, was an undervalued subject at home and at school. Even the honor of being elected head of the Drama Society carried no credit, although the position prepared me for the world of fashion magazines far more than algebra or Latin did. In one dramatic role, as the warden of a women's prison, I got to wear seamed stockings (which did not go unnoticed by audience members from the Boys' College). Our senior play was *Salad Days*, about some people who find a magic talking piano that leads them around the world. I was thrilled to be voted in as producer, and became set designer, makeup artist, and wardrobe mistress, also playing a sexy nightclub singer in a dress of purple skirt-lining fabric I made myself. After the performance (a huge success; I'm surprised you never heard about it), my friend Libby Mills and I climbed to the top of the Worcester Beacons, the hills behind the school, to lie in tall grass and drink a whole bottle of champagne that we'd managed to steal from home. Despite our pseudo-sophistication, we hadn't a clue how to pop the cork and were rescued (and joined) by a passing boy on a hike.

I was called "Kelly Bonks" at school (I no longer have any idea what the "Bonks" part conveyed, although it had nothing to do with sexual "bonking"). My gang was known as a pretty wild lot, especially after lights out, when we might listen to pirated Radio Luxembourg under the bedcovers or climb out the windows for nocturnal visits to another dorm. I slept in hair rollers every night despite the fact that we were not permitted to date. I quickly learned the crucial differentiation between what was "in" (Elvis, the Beatles, coffee bars) and what was "out" ("10 to 100" dances, where youngsters were expected to dance with their senescent parents). I also learned compassion and respect. Living with adolescent girls in the close quarters of a dorm, I got drawn in to the intimate details of lives in transition—when they got their first period or first boyfriend, when their dog or grandmother died. If somebody was crying in the corridor, I had to put my arm around her. I had to be courteous to seniors and kind to juniors, even if I didn't feel like it. Some people were prigs, and I came to despise their parochial thinking and self-absorption. The experience taught me that people's feelings count, that they don't have to conform to my standards of right and wrong, that if I make enough effort, I'll find something pleasing under the skin of the most disagreeable character.

Sports was my metier. I played left defense in lacrosse and left wing in hockey, and I played fast and rough—I pushed my opponents, tripped them up, broke noses. On weekends, my parents would come to games on fields frozen solid and covered in hoarfrost, huddling for warmth on the sidelines. After the game we'd sit in the car eating cupcakes and drinking tea out of thermos bottles, my father moaning about fair play and sportsmanship. "Elizabeth," he'd admonish, "you are fierce."

Yes, I am. People who think of me as smiling, saintly Liz aren't getting the whole measure of my lacrosse-stick-wielding capabilities, which are still with me, popping up from time to time. Years later, while I was editor of British *Vogue*, I was at a Jean-Paul Gaultier show in Paris. It was raining, there were huge lakes of mud, and a frightening crush of people tried jostling and squashing each other to gain entrance. A security guard pushed one of my editors off a walkway into a puddle, and I slugged him. By the time I got back to the London office, the staff had hung a banner over my door saying "Welcome Home, Mrs. T" with a drawing of Chanel boxing gloves.

As the weather got warm, I'd slather myself with olive oil and lie out on the school lawn to get a tan (the initials SPF had not yet entered anyone's vocabulary) and spend summer vacations with my family, visiting every single cathedral and museum from Rheims to Rome. My father would get an idea in his head, and we'd all cram in the car for another eccentric journey. Once he tied a mahogany diving board to the roof of the car so he could drill it into a rock in Ischia. Because our plans were haphazard and impromptu, nothing ever went smoothly. We were always ending up in a stalled car on an unpaved road with a river pouring over it and no place to spend the night. We usually picnicked by the roadside, but if we wanted to splurge on a proper restaurant meal, that was my department. It was amazing how the best table at a French brasserie or a Spanish nightclub would suddenly materialize for an English teenager wearing a miniskirt. Then, before the darling Latin busboys could make any arrangements to meet me at closing time, my father would whisk us away.

British students in my day were required to compete in two rounds of standardized tests: "O" (ordinary) levels at around age sixteen, and "A" (advanced) levels at around eighteen. "A" levels were more specialized and, depending on the results, were meant to indicate the future profession one could aim for. My A-level grades were a sure indication of my talents and weaknesses: A in art, C in history, E in Spanish. Despite my academic deficiency, as graduation approached my parents hatched the idea that I go live with Cousin Isabel in Mexico City and, like her, become an anthropologist. It was an imprudent proposal if I intended to *speak* with anyone while living there—as my grade in Spanish indicated, I have no aptitude for any language beyond that of the land of my birth, and the notion of memorizing whether a noun is masculine or feminine makes me want to stoop and kiss English soil—but I dutifully started the rounds of interviews at every university that had a Spanish program. I also brought along a large portfolio of watercolors and oils and screen prints. The admissions officers would take one look at my drawings of women in historically correct Victorian dress and ask, "Why aren't you applying for art school?" I couldn't say, "Well brought up girls don't go to art school, because their parents will think them failures." The mailbox filled up with rejections.

That summer after graduation, unsure of my future, I enrolled in a secretarial course at the state-funded technical college in the beautiful Georgian city of Bath, where my parents had moved in 1959 when my father became a consultant at the Royal Eye Infirmary there. We lived in a huge hundred-year-old sandstone house called Linden (in those days, the bigger the house was, the cheaper), next to the Priory Hotel, with my father's consulting rooms on the ground floor and his secretary working at our kitchen table.

Daddy had a mania for swimming pools—we'd always had one of those inexpensive circular things—and at Linden he decided to built an in-ground pool, but there were no bulldozers available, so we dug it ourselves with shovels. My father designed the plastic liner and the solar panels to heat it—the height of improbability (or optimism) in Britain. One rainy day, when the vinyl had been installed and Daddy was walking down the slope of the pool to inspect it, he slipped and was knocked unconscious. I'd learned lifesaving at school, so I jumped in and started performing mouth-to-mouth resuscitation, interspersed with banshee screams to fetch the doctor at the top of the hill. My startled father came around to find his teenage daughter holding his nose and giving him the kiss of life. But the experience didn't taint his enthusiasm for the pool, even when we had to carry endless kettles of hot water down the lawn to heat it.

My parents turned the basement level of the house over to the kids, and my first boyfriend, Simon Byrne, was the drummer in a band that rehearsed there and played every weekend. That summer was one long party, my first taste of freedom. At the annual Bath Festival, even the royal family came to swim in the Roman baths

61

and eat ancient delicacies like fried field mice. Such a busy social calendar meant I had a constant need for new clothes, so I got into dressmaking, working on a sewing machine with a hand winder to produce my own versions of the Carnaby Street look: halternecks and minis, worn with fishnet tights and long dangly earrings, black eyeliner, and matte white lipstick—a poor man's Mary Quant. Then Simon dumped me, heartlessly turning up at a party with another girl who was a brilliant horsewoman. When I recovered, I started dating Tom Borthwick, an artist I'd met at the Tech, and we hung out in pubs and clubs, where everyone competed to stay out the latest and dance the longest. My parents didn't approve of my dating an artist with long floppy hair, but there were no drugs around, at least in our crowd. Drugs were the playthings of the rich.

My family finally got the message that their eldest child was not going to work in any respectable field of endeavor, and once I started interviewing at art schools, I was accepted by four or five of the best in Britain and was spoiled for choice. A little research revealed that Leicester Polytechnic had a good fashion design course, and by the time we set out for our summer holiday in Germany, my educational future was decided. But my personal future was in abeyance. It was the year before the birth-control pill became available in the United Kingdom. And at just eighteen, I realized I was pregnant.

I spent that trip in a tortured state of anxiety and shame, lying in bed and beating on my stomach in an attempt to miscarry, unable to contemplate the idea of having a child. When we got home, I told no one but my boyfriend, Tom, who started making frantic inquiries about abortions, still illegal unless pregnancy jeopardized the physical or mental health of the mother. Every morning I'd agonize in front of the mirror to see whether I "showed" yet, and every night I'd cry to Tom about the ruination of my plans and very likely my life. Finally he found a contact in London, and we scraped together 120 pounds, about $200, from our savings accounts. To comply with the law, I needed the signatures of two psychiatrists, whom I met in gloomy basement offices in London—

perfunctory meetings where I was asked, "Are you depressed, anxious, scared, confused?" Tom was coming in on the train from Bath to take me to the clinic in Edgware, at the end of the Bakerloo subway line. We'd traveled separately to the city so that our being out of town together wouldn't arouse suspicion with our parents. But somehow I missed him at the station and ended up sobbing to myself all the way to the clinic. I'd never known anyone who'd had an abortion, and I'd never even been treated by anyone but our local GP or my own father.

Few doctors performed abortions in those days, and they weren't necessarily trained ob/gyns. When I arrived at the clinic, I learned that I was to be attended by an eye surgeon who knew my father and had called him to inform him of his daughter's activities. To his everlasting credit, Daddy gave his permission for the procedure and promised to collect me from the clinic the next day. I awoke from anesthesia on the operating table with my legs still in stirrups, the pain deep inside like the worst kind of cramps multiplied a hundredfold. Tom never did get there, and I saw no one else except nurses. But I accidentally walked into a room where I caught a glimpse of slop buckets filled with bloody water before a nurse yelled, "You're not permitted in there!" and yanked me back by force.

The decision to end that pregnancy was not a moral dilemma for me: I believed then and now that children should be born to mature, capable parents, and that an embryo is the *possibility* of life, not a human being. (The English theater director and physician Jonathan Miller expresses this idea with perfect clarity: "Anyone who contends that the living sperm has a right to life might wish to say a requiem mass every time he takes a hot bath.") In the years to come, I never thought of my infertility as some divine retribution or quid pro quo for my earlier decision to terminate a pregnancy. But although it was surely a more common occurrence in the British upper classes than anyone would admit, and although my father knew the facts of life about unwanted pregnancy from a physician's firsthand vantage point, my abortion certainly sent shock waves through my genteel family. There was no scene, no histrionics—we were all too polite for that. My father let me sleep most of the trip home, only inquiring after my comfort and well-being. My mother brought me cups of tea but never spoke to me about the abortion at all, not that day or ever afterward.

Starting at Leicester Polytechnic in the fall of 1965, I had barely got in before I was thrown out. Social mores were changing irrevocably, and a family planning clinic had just been established in town, but if the sexual revolution was taking place, it had not reached the principal of my college. About three weeks into the term, I broke curfew and nearly broke my neck shinnying down the drainpipe to see Tom, and I decided not to risk it again. The next night, he came up to my room. But I forgot that the housemistress lived directly below me. She heard some suspicious noises and burst in on us, drinking blue cider and just shy of in flagrante delicto. I was hauled off to the principal, who sputtered "How dare you?" a few times before expelling me.

My parents had gotten quite used to saying, "Oh, Elizabeth." I did what I wanted with scant regard for public opinion or possible consequences, and obviously I was destined to be no good. But I loved fashion with such ardor that nothing so inconsequential as shame and infamy would make me give it up. If I was to continue the academic year, I'd have to go somewhere else. I was still following the "pre-diploma" program, wherein students got a little sampling of courses (sculpture, fine arts, textile and industrial design) before selecting a field of concentration. The head of the pre-dip at Leicester, Derek Carruthers, thought that my expulsion based on an outdated moral code was absurd and that I was good enough to deserve a second chance. He had a friend at the Jacob Kramer Art College in Leeds in the north of England, where I could finish my year's pre-diploma course, and I had a school friend whose family made biscuits there. So I turned up, quaking, to be interviewed, and the first person who looked at my portfolio was Andrew Tilberis.

The son of a Greek restaurateur, Andrew had attended St. Martin's School of Art in London and worked as a TV set designer and architectural assistant, showing his own paintings at several exhibitions while still a student, including "The Young Con-temporaries" in 1961 and 1962, alongside David Hockney, Ron Kitaj, and Patrick Proctor. Later, he made and exhibited "struc-turist" works of art, a movement started by the American Charles Biederman. In defiance of the prevailing trends of abstract expressionism and pop art, structurists maintained that art had to have a real structure developed through the study of nature and that artists had to know about color, light, and space. I knew Andrew was hardly likely to be impressed by the dilettante efforts of a posh ex-boarding school girl, and the one-eyed principal of the school, appalled by the offense that had got me expelled from Leicester, tried to block my admission, saying, "We don't want any hookers here." But I was determined to overwhelm them with my enthusiasm for fashion: why I loved it, why it was important, why I needed the chance to study it. Andrew says it was that little speech that allowed my academic career to continue. That . . . and my legs.

Once I arrived in Leeds, it became obvious that Andrew was a ladies' man—"Beware the Greek" was the reputation that preceded him. He was an artist, he drove a Porsche 356sc, he knew about judo and jazz, he wore elegant Ivy League clothes when other young men were sporting brocade turtlenecks and purple velvet bell-bottoms. I was living at the local YWCA, and my window looked diagonally onto Andrew's apartment, where I could observe an endless line of long-haired, miniskirted colleagues trooping up and down his stairs and standing at the sink to wash his socks. I was used to well-mannered doctors' sons, and Andrew was a rebel with a cause. Relationships between teachers and students were strictly forbidden, even though Andrew was only five years my senior, but I was determined to get him to notice me. My moment came one lunchtime when I went with a girlfriend to Whitelocks Pub, an Edwardian saloon that sparkled with refracted light from mirrors and etched glass. As we sat down on a banquette, Andrew happened to be sitting opposite me. I looked straight into his eyes. I was wearing a black turtleneck, patent sling-backs, and a mustard thigh-high mini. He noticed.

Somehow we managed to keep our affair a secret—otherwise, he certainly would have been fired, and I could have been expelled for a second and probably final time. But we weren't recluses. Andrew had no interest in the Beatles or the Rolling Stones—he took me to hear Duke Ellington, Otis Redding, Sam and Dave, West Indian bluebeat and ska, and we were often the only white people in the place. One night my purse was stolen from a club, and Andrew enlisted the help of a friend who called himself Headhunter, a huge black man with bloodshot eyes, smoking a joint. He put the word out, and my purse was back in ten minutes. (Headhunter is now an important person in the Congo.) Since Andrew was obsessed with sports cars, I considered it my duty to accompany him to motor races—once we traveled by charter bus to the twenty-four-hour races at Le Mans, where it rained for twenty-three of the hours and we had to sleep on the bus. (As soon as we got married, I felt these duties were over, but the Porsches kept coming, as did our rows about their cost.) Sometimes we went camping—on one trip to Spain, the nearest campground was at the foot of the Barcelona Airport runway, where we had to hang on to the tent poles in a rainstorm, with the planes taking off overhead. It wasn't always my idea of a good time, but it was never boring, and it was a great letdown when my year's "disgrace" was over and I returned to Leicester, sharing a terraced Victorian house with three other girls. (My room in the gables was painted sludge green by my friend Charles Dance, who was studying industrial design long before he starred in *The Jewel in the Crown*.) That year in Leeds confirmed two things: my passion for fashion and my passion for Andrew.

The late 1960s was an amazing time to be young, English, and studying fashion. The miniskirt might have been born in Paris, fathered by André Courrèges, but we Brits had usurped the lead in the fashion sweepstakes. The best clothes were ours, and they were for the young, the skinny, and the hip. Styles were in and out in a week, and we didn't care who we shocked. Twiggy was launched as "the face of the year" in 1966, a ninety-pound Cockney waif with her hair chopped into a boyish crop by the society hairdresser Leonard, whose chic Mayfair salon backed onto the American embassy. Mick Jagger, Marianne Faithfull, Yoko Ono, and Mia Farrow shopped at Biba for big-brimmed hats, skimpy dresses, colorful tights, stretchy bras, and feather boas. Mary Quant went to Buckingham Palace in a miniskirt and cut-away gloves to receive the Order of the British Empire from the queen.

In 1968, a teen magazine called *Petticoat/Trend* came to Leicester to find "groovy chicks" and discovered, among others, one Liz Kelly. I was photographed standing on a wall, hands on hips, a Bonnie and Clyde wannabe, in black leather knee-high boots, a double-breasted tweed maxi-coat, a red beret, and my long brown hair over one eye. The coat was made by Bus Stop and cost 8 pounds, 18 shillings and sixpence. It's almost identical to what Prada is doing today. (The photo caption read, "Liz Kelly likes giving parties in her flat, so she's permanently broke. At the moment she desperately needs a chest of drawers, so please send donations!")

That was my one and only shot at modeling. But as I moved into my final year at Leicester, I realized I wasn't going to be a designer either. I could swing a bust dart like a pro, but designing takes something more: patience, originality, conceptual skills, and clear, uncomplicated thinking. The best designs in the world are the plainest. A designer has to look at an inert bolt of fabric and see a strapless ballgown or a peplum jacket. I'm in awe of anyone who can make the translation from a dress pattern, which is made of floppy brown cardboard, to an exquisite finished piece. I was interested in how fashion looks and changes. I didn't care about making the garment, but I reveled in the finished product—the cut, the drape, the optical effect of fabrics and what they would do, what was surprising, how luxury was defined and redefined. The difference between being a fashion designer and a fashion editor may be the difference between cooking and eating. Editing is appreciation and application. Thanks to my art school training, I was beginning to see the excitement of fashion photography, layout, the whole packaging of a look. My final thesis was "The

Development of a Fashion Journal," and the first page was ... the cover of a 1914 *Harper's Bazaar*.

The only major fashion magazine in Britain then was *Vogue*, which was held for me every month at the local news agent. I could smell those pages. The bright, clean-cut, space-age vision of the early sixties was turning into something far more whimsical, decorative, and allusive, an outrageous fantasy phase. Part of it was the visual expression of the dropout aesthetic, the counterculture fueled by hallucinogenic drugs. I was enthralled with the look of it, but the drugs themselves simply passed me by. Despite my rebellious nature, I was not interested in a high any more dangerous and mind-blowing than could be obtained at the local pub, supplemented by the occasional joint with Andrew's arty friends. I guess I like my own equilibrium and sense of control.

One day my roommate Avril Hiley and I went to the local café for our usual lunch of eggs and chips (all fried, of course), poring over our new copy of *Vogue* as we ate. Avril was amazingly stylish and ballsy. If anybody was going to wear a feather boa, it was she. Her standard garb was boots, then a massive stretch of leg and the tiniest bit of fabric that could legally be called a skirt. She was chatty, confident, chain-smoking, with red hair and freckles, like a flapper from the Roaring Twenties. "Hey," she said, leafing through the pages of our bible, "there's a talent contest. Let's do it." The entrance requirement was three brief essays, including one about an influential person in fashion, and the winner would be offered a summer internship at the magazine. Avril lost her initial enthusiasm, but I got started right away, choosing to write about the costume historian James Laver. It was from his work that I'd learned how fashion is connected to the wider world, that hemlines predict societal shifts, that voluminous quantities of fabric and tarted-up designs can be an antidote to an economic slump, whereas fashion simplicity often reflects economic security. I also illustrated a wardrobe of my own design—pantsuit, ballgown, suit, and dress—the drawings backed on pale turquoise cards.

Just after the spring term ended, I was thrilled to get a letter notifying me that I was a finalist and inviting me to join Beatrix

Miller, the editor-in-chief, some senior staff, and guest judges for luncheon at Vogue House, the magazine's offices in Hanover Square. I panicked: Obviously my choice of outfit would figure in the judges' deliberations, and I simply didn't have any money. Finally I found a chic Polly Peck black wool jersey pantsuit on sale. As a good luck charm, I bought an expensive chiffon scarf printed by Celia Birtwell (who was married to the late designer Ossie Clark and frequently posed for David Hockney). Celia's distinctive floral design would, I felt certain, signal that I was among the fashion cognoscenti.

Six round tables and gold chairs were set up in the boardroom on the fourth floor at Vogue House for the twenty finalists and half a dozen celebrity judges. I kept trying not to stare at Peter Sellers and Lord Snowdon, but I'd never before been in the same room with anyone so glamorous and famous. While I was endeavoring to be witty and clever, the waiter set before me a dish that was a nightmare to eat gracefully: spaghetti with spinach on the side— probably a "pop quiz" to test an entrant's table manners and thereby discern her breeding. I didn't think I had a chance, but I must have conveyed my ardor for fashion, and by the time I called my parents from the platform at Paddington Station on my way home, the results had been announced. "We've just had a telegram!" my mother yelled. "You're the runner-up, darling!" The winner, an art student at Sussex University, turned down the internship to continue her studies, and I was offered her place. Two hours later, when I walked into my parents' house straight off the train, I was greeted by a press photographer. My proud father had called the local newspaper, the *Bath and Wiltshire Evening Chronicle*, and the next day, Wednesday, April 23, 1969, I was front-page news, wearing my prized scarf and chewing a pen in what I thought was a journalistic pose. The *Chronicle* offered me my first paid job in fashion, writing a column about styles and trends called "Live Wire" for 5 pounds a week. From British *Vogue* I'd won a whopping 25 pounds, plus a year's subscription, and the first step in a career that took me all the way.

# 5

STEPPING INTO THE elevator on my first day as an intern that summer, I saw one of the *Vogue* editors in the same raincoat I was wearing. But hers was real patent leather from Harvey Nichols, the smart store favored by the well-born young women who came to be known as Sloane Rangers, and mine was a plastic knockoff from the Soho Market. It was an omen. For a long time, I would try to be chic on a shoestring, competing with the smartest pack of women I had ever seen.

Sheila Wetton, the fashion director, had been a model for Molyneux in the 1930s and 1940s. She wore her graying hair in an impeccable chignon and dressed with the sort of cashmere-and-pearls elegance that is the epitome of English good taste, but she swore like a sailor on shore leave. "Another fucking camel coat!" she'd fume, and I'd wonder how any garment could evoke such fury. She had a rapier wit and could be hilariously funny. The receptionist once called our department to report some men wearing burnooses in the lobby. Sheila put her hand over the phone and asked, "Did anyone order any Arabs?" She must have been a devastating beauty in her youth, and we got the impression that she'd had a pretty good time during the London blitz, living in a garret during those inhibition-freeing days when soldiers were returning to the front and young people never knew whether they'd live to see tomorrow.

At *Vogue* Sheila was responsible for the "p-and-s" pages, the "pure and simple" clothes that gave the magazine its ladylike backbone: the Norfolk jackets, Fair Isle cardigans, twills and tweeds that readers in the English provinces could really wear. It was all done with a certain sophisticated style—not Queen Elizabeth's frumpy librarian look—but those classic clothes weren't quite fashion-forward enough for us, so the "p-and-s" pages were known in-house as "piss-and-shit."

Not to be upstaged in the fashion department was Grace Coddington. Amazing Grace, as her epithet went, had been modeling since 1959, often for *Vogue*, and I can say without the prejudice of friendship that she was one of the greats, not in terms of mere beauty but because of the interpretative powers that enabled her to engage in the photographs on a level few models ever reach. Her face and posture could reflect haughty insolence, mischievous decadence, or serene come-hitherness, and her chameleon looks had expressed the myriad phases of fashion so successfully, you often had to look twice at a photo to check whether or not it was her. Grace's unusual appearance was more than the average gift from God: When she was just starting out as a model, still waitressing at the Chelsea Potter, her eyelid had been sheared off in a car accident and a new lid was crafted out of a flap of skin taken from under her arm. It gave her a wonderful individuality in photographs, because her face is not perfectly symmetrical. Sheila had spotted Grace's exceptional taste and understanding of photography, and recruited her to join the staff of *Vogue* as a fashion editor when she was ready to quit modeling in 1968, but right up until the early 1970s she was still getting into the photos—like Hitchcock in his films, she'd just turn up. One of her last jobs in front of the camera was a sexually charged session with Helmut Newton, the voyeuristic, taboo-breaking German photographer, shot after dark in a swimming pool, with Grace in a black bikini, red nail polish, and some kinky harlequin sunglasses.

To outsiders, Grace was and still is an enigma—elusive, severe, silent. If she rates you as someone who understands fashion, the beautiful statue becomes animated, and you are drowned in an eloquent runaway monologue about the color purple or a pinstripe. But if Grace dismisses you as unworthy of her commentary, you might as well be part of the wallpaper. This air of detachment and the impact of her presence as a fashion icon make her terrifying, even to this day. Tall and slim, with the longest legs I've ever seen, she could transform her personal style thoroughly and instantaneously—flowing robes would be replaced almost overnight by sculptural Yves Saint Laurent pantsuits, her long red hair suddenly chopped off and dyed punk blond—and it was guaranteed that any new look, no matter how radical and unimaginable, was a premonition of the next fashion wave, that a year down the road, everyone would be wearing it. Grace was the first person I ever saw wearing hot pants, and she wore bra tops under sheer net shirts long before Madonna.

When we met, she was in her "hippie deluxe" moment. The first time I worked for her, she was wearing a djellaba, her red hair short and twisted under a turban, on her way to a sitting. ("Sitting" is *Vogue*-speak for a photo shoot, an old-fashioned term that dates back, I think, to the earliest days of society photography when subjects literally sat for a portrait.) She was married at the time to Michael Chow, who was introducing gourmet Chinese food at the original branch of his restaurant chain Mr. Chow's. We drove in their beige convertible Rolls-Royce, with Schubert playing on the radio, down Park Lane past the Dorchester and other fabled hostelries to Marble Arch. I was twenty-one years old, living like a mouse with Andrew's parents in the North London community of Child's Hill, and I thought that if I was hit by a bus the next day, I'd lived a full life, needing no further thrill or compensation. Miss Elizabeth Kelly had arrived.

At Vogue House, one took a hard left out of the elevators on the fifth floor for the fashion department, which consisted of red wooden desks for five editors and their assistants, with Royal Standard typewriters (the kind where you had to punch the keys down several inches and use tweezers to change the ribbon), and a bulletin board over each desk. The rule was: only one boyfriend picture allowed per board. What we kept there were fabric samples, phone numbers, head sheets from model agencies, and favorite fashion shots. The clothes were stored on rolling racks in a room-size "closet," with other closets for hats, shoes, gloves, and accessories. Each assistant had a locker in the fashion closet to store anything that might be needed at a sitting: scissors, Scotch tape, hair dryer, Tampax. Assistants were expected to provide assistance, whatever that might mean. Even as an intern, I started to book the models and make travel arrangements for out-of-town locations, but I went only to local sittings around London or in the *Vogue* studios, up one flight of stairs on the sixth floor. I was responsible for packing the clothes in suitcases and ironing them when they came out, fetching ice cream when it was hot and tea when it was cold. I started out picking up pins and graduated to sewing on buttons. I made sure that the model had her tissues, her Marlboros, her boyfriend's phone number.

*Vogue* at that time was like a finishing school. The editorial offices were liberally populated with the daughters of the aristocracy and the socially connected rich: young women with double-barreled surnames, dating young men whom I associated with streets and counties in Britain—Wiltons and Somersets and Grosvenors. Their manners often reflected the social dynamics of their terribly proper families: the class consciousness, the competitiveness, the capacity for bitchiness that is cemented at public school, where girls learn to be interested in other people in order to get information out of them, to dismiss them if they're not useful or important. There was much talk about who was dating Prince Charles or Paul McCartney, who had fallen off a horse while riding to hounds, who was afraid she might be pregnant, who was trying to get married, who was trying to get divorced, whose belligerent boyfriend got his kicks by slapping women around. Those first cups of morning coffee were *exhausting*—we could have employed

73

the full-time services of a resident gynecologist and psychiatrist. There was a lot of crying in the bathrooms, and sometimes it was being done by me. These people were going out to glamorous dinners and dances, and I was going home to Andrew's family. One of the glamour girls married the Duke of Westminster. Another visited prisons on weekends, part of the noblesse oblige for someone of her station. We were given lunch vouchers worth 20 pence a day, about 50 cents, and one girl blew a whole month's packet on a single meal, an extravagance that left me speechless.

There was a certain Darwinian atmosphere to the office. An assistant needed finely tuned antennae to work out a place in the vaguely defined chain of command, and then she had two choices: Do nothing much and eventually disappear into marriage, or do as I did, making myself useful and, slowly, very slowly, working my way up. In hindsight, although never by schematic design, I think I succeeded at *Vogue* by knowing when to keep my mouth shut, when to smile, and how to do really, really good ironing. I was a bundle of enthusiasm and energy, naive and inexperienced, but I'd also learned everything there was to know about the way fabric behaves—how to press crepe de chine (there was a lot of it around in those days) or get a spot out of silk or keep jersey from stretching—and the training gave me a jump on the other "juniors."

If *Vogue* was a school, the headmistress was Beatrix Miller, the upright, elegant, and formidable editor-in-chief, always addressed as "Miss Miller." (I only received permission to call her Bea about twenty years later and would always choke on it.) Out of earshot, she was Queen Bea (she had been the editor of *Queen* magazine for five years). She had an ample bosom, a round Teutonic face, short, curly blond hair and was usually dressed in the muted chic of her friend Jean Muir. Although I knew her long and well, eventually as a peer invited to her home for parties that featured masses of white flowers and a butler serving cold pea soup, I never had an inkling about her personal life, if there was one. She was a woman devoted to her career, with no mention of a significant other, and none of us would have dared ask, not even the senior staff.

Miss Miller had nicknames for people and inanimate objects, driving to work in a large white Jaguar that she called Arctic. British *Vogue* itself was dubbed *Brogue* to differentiate it from its American counterpart, where Miss Miller had worked at the beginning of her career. Every morning an assistant brought her a vitamin C tablet and sometimes replacement stockings from Marks and Spencer. (*Everyone* in London, even the editor of *Vogue*, patronized the famous mass-market chain store affectionately known as Marks and Sparks.) Then she proceeded to write all of her appointments, phone messages, and ideas in blue ink on the top sheet of a large desk blotter, ripping it off at the end of the day for her secretary to transcribe.

Miss Miller staged revolutions. She'd stride down the corridor, hands on hips, pointing and declaring, "Today is a revolution." She would change all the sections of the magazine, or all the layouts, or all the models, just to shake everyone up and get their creative juices going. She derived great glee from doing it, with a lovely smile on her face. Encountering her in that mode was petrifying but rather glamorous, as it was generally the only contact such a junior person would have. "I always used to pee at the same time as Miss Miller," one assistant recalled later. "I took it as an auspicious sign."

For all her starchy correctness, Miss Miller was not a prude and had an extraordinary knack for bringing personalities into the magazine who reflected the racy and decadent glamour of the decade. It was the time of "the beautiful people," of Astors and Agnellis and the Aga Khan jetting off to Costa Smeralda and Chamonix. In London the scene was concentrated around a nucleus of actors, singers, designers, models, and exquisite-looking young aristocrats. Pictured in the magazine were Omar Sharif, Jacqueline Bisset, Baron Guy de Rothschild, Princess Grace of Monaco, Christina Onassis, the Michaels (Caine and York), the heart surgeon Christiaan Barnard, and, of course, Richard Burton and Elizabeth Taylor. Opening the pages of *Vogue* was like being invited to the best party that never really happened, an editorially enhanced social mix of the most influential, creative, patrician, and exotic people.

Miss Miller loved the royals and was certainly prepared to hold back an issue from the printers in order to get in photos of some duke or viscount's wedding. (*Vogue* reported the marriage of Camilla Shand to Andrew Parker-Bowles in 1973, with photographs of the Queen Mother and Princess Anne as guests, although Prince Charles is nowhere to be seen.) Sometimes Miss Miller had the inside track: Her own secretary was Sarah Spencer, who had dated Prince Charles before she married landowner Neil McCorquodale (and before her little sister Diana came on the scene). The other Spencer sister, Jane, worked for the beauty editor, Felicity Clark, and subsequently married the queen's private secretary, the Right Honorable Sir Robert Fellowes.

The fashion pages were a bit schizophrenic in those days. There were the queen and her sister and daughter looking like ... well, you know what they looked like. British *Vogue* could never sacrifice the sensibilities of the middle-class, middle-aged reader who admired and emulated that frumpy upper-class style, and the p-and-s pages paid proper homage to the shirtwaist dresses, Burberry raincoats, and tweedy suits that a dowager duchess might wear. But it was the pulsating energy of music, film, and art that was the lifeblood of fashion. Rock stars and their girlfriends were beauty icons: Patti Boyd, the wide-eyed girl who was to break George Harrison's heart, was a *Vogue* supermodel (although the word hadn't been invented yet), with a languid sensuality that made her perfect for underwear stories. I bumped into Bianca Jagger in the elevator, not long after she'd married Mick, looking like a fictional dandy in a Saint Laurent white tuxedo with a hat and cane.

Lee Radziwill, Anjelica Huston, Geraldine Chaplin, Marisa Berenson, Julie Christie, and Charlotte Rampling all appeared as models. There were a lot of "before" pictures: Britt Ekland before she married Peter Sellers, Ann Turkel before she married Richard Harris, Victoria Tennant before she married Steve Martin, Bonnie Pfeiffer before she married Gene Pressman, the president of Barneys, Lyndall Hobbs before she was attached to Al Pacino, Joanna Lumley before she became "Absolutely Fabulous." (The magazine editor she portrays in that show is said to be an amalgam of various *Vogue* employees, all of whom she knew as a model.) The *Vogue* "Living" section captured fascinating people in their private habitats: Saint Laurent himself, slim-hipped, long-haired, and leather-clad on his ivory terrace in Marrakech; or the sculptor Allen Jones at home with his outrageous furniture made from plastic models of women in S&M boots and underwear. British *Vogue* described the defining youth event of 1970, the Isle of Wight Festival—Britain's answer to Woodstock—as something "from Satyricon out of Mary Poppins." It was clear that the clothes, the music, the happenings were all part of the same thing: Youth culture had fused with high style.

I was deliriously happy to be a part of this scene, even at the lowest level. I never had the slightest idea about or interest in the editing of a fashion magazine. All I cared about was being able to hand Jean Shrimpton a pair of shoes. (At the height of her reign, the beautiful six-foot-one "Shrimp" became disenchanted with modeling and went off to the English countryside to become surely the world's most glamorous innkeeper.) My revelation came when, as a mere intern, I was allowed to help the editor Melanie Miller on an important sitting with the top models Penelope Tree and Maudie James, photographed by the wonderfully innovative but terrifyingly perfectionistic Guy Bourdin. I was running in and out of the studio with the clothes—flimsy, reckless frippery by Thea Porter and Chloé—helping to adjust little sequined skullcaps and mile-long strands of pearls, unrolling the white paper called no-seam, hung from a huge tube in the ceiling, that provided a clean backdrop. I saw what makes a good model: She knows the capability of the clothes, knows when to blink and how to exercise her mouth so she can keep smiling. As she walks across the no-seam and turns to the camera—not once, not twice, but a hundred times—the belt will be tight and the coat will be flowing, and her body will be adjusted just so for a thinner silhouette at the hips.

From then on, I knew what a real fashion shoot should be like—and that it was the only thing in the world I wanted to do. I understood the synergy and lyricism and choreography of collecting the most dazzling clothes, the most beautiful models, the

77

most assured photographer, the most creative hairdressers and makeup artists. It was all about *the most*, about the visuals of that moment in fashion being recorded for posterity at the highest level of quality, about seeing the combination of elements on a woman's body instead of a hanger, about the way the lighting accentuated everything that was supposed to be accentuated. The minute I saw it happening, I wanted to do it and knew I could. I *would* be a fashion editor one day. I was to learn that it's actually quite difficult and more complicated than I realized because of the politics and problems behind the scenes—which photographer is sleeping with which model, which model doesn't show up because she's been partying too hard, which designer is making silhouettes so boring or repetitive or unflattering that the only thing to do is an artist's sketch (more flexible about flaws than a photograph). But it felt as natural to me as putting on a sweater when I was cold.

Toward the end of my three-month internship, Grace Coddington's assistant announced that she was leaving and recommended me as a replacement. I had a heartbreaking decision. *Vogue* had felt like a homecoming to me, and I desperately wanted a permanent place there, but I still had one more year of college to complete to get my B.A. When Grace offered me the job, she was in a dressing room on the studio floor completing a sitting. I took a deep breath. "My parents have invested so much in my college education," I explained. "I can't let them down. But would you have me back when I've graduated?" Grace must have been shocked—it was unheard-of to turn down such an offer and try to put the job on hold—but she didn't show it. "I respect your decision," she said. "Call when you've graduated." And I left the world of sequins and pearls for the smokestacks of Leicester.

ANDREW WAS STILL living in Leeds, the two of us commuting to see each other on weekends either in Leeds or London. One Sunday while I was cooking breakfast in his tiny kitchen, he called to me from the bed, "I've been thinking we should get married."

I burned a hole in the frying pan, and nearly torched the apartment, while I ran in to hug him. Andrew seemed to take this as a yes. "Right," he said. "Then that's that. But how do we handle your father?" Andrew was only too well aware of my father's narrow-mindedness about nationality and class. No Greek would have been good enough for me—oh, perhaps a rich Greek or a royal Greek, but certainly not an arty Greek or, worse, a restaurant Greek.

My parents were coming up to Leicester to see my diploma show. In order to get my degree, I had to produce a collection of clothes—draw them, cut the patterns, sew or knit them, get them photographed, and mount them for display. A friend of Andrew's named Bill Major agreed to photograph the clothes, a group of dresses in a Liberty fabric of cotton lawn with tiny florals, and I mounted a group of my "Live Wire" columns. I got a grade of "upper second"—not a first, but pretty good—and to celebrate, my parents took Andrew and me out to dinner. We decided that was the moment to broach the subject of marriage. Over coffee, Andrew said, "Tom, I've got something to talk about with you." My father suddenly looked like thunder—he knew what was coming—but he quashed any further discussion at that moment by loudly demanding the check and heading for the car. When we arrived at my apartment, I fled inside with my mother while Andrew cornered Daddy in the car and formally, calmly, and properly asked for my hand in marriage.

"I've got no money, you know," my father rejoined.

"I know that," said Andrew, "and I'll take care of Liz."

"I don't want her marrying a foreigner," came my father's retort.

"I am British," Andrew said calmly. "I don't wish to break up your family, but Liz and I have decided to get married, with or without your permission. We'll set a date and wait one year so you can get used to the idea. But on that day, we're getting married."

Daddy had one parting shot. "If you marry Elizabeth," he said, "she'll never be successful." Andrew had sweet revenge reminding him of that dire prediction twenty years later, when I became editor of British *Vogue*. By that time, my husband and my father had thrashed out all their differences and become drinking buddies. But right up until our wedding, Daddy acted like it wasn't happening, completely ignoring all the preparations. When he went to bed on the eve of the ceremony, he refused to let me kiss him good night, and as we drove to the registrar's office with my bridesmaids on our wedding day, July 17, 1971, he was babbling about the intricate workings of the limousine's engine, still unable to face what was happening.

In July 1970 I had started as an assistant at *Vogue*, but not to Grace, who hadn't been able to wait a year for me. My bosses were Mandy Clapperton and Sandy Boler-Hamilton, who was pregnant with her first child and was soon to be replaced by Polly Hamilton. (Polly now works for Donna Karan. Sandy now edits British *Bride's* magazine.) I worked very happily as an assistant for a year, and began preparations for my wedding, which, as planned, was to be held a year after we had announced our engagement.

One of the girls at work, the one who blew all her luncheon vouchers in one fell swoop, went to a sample sale at Jean Muir one day and came back to say, "I've found your wedding dress." I bought it on the spot for 30 pounds: a midcalf, cream-colored, satin-backed crepe jersey, with a pin-tucked bodice and rouleaux fabric buttons, worn with matching wedge sandals I dyed myself. For my going-away outfit, I chose a pair of white cotton trousers and a blue satin blazer with red buttons, made by Sheridan Barnett for a company called Copper Coin.

My wedding must have been quite a spectacle for any residents of Bath who may have been passing by the registry office: my frightfully proper English relations in top hats and tails; the *Vogue* lot, in extravagant printed Kenzo dresses, with plastic cherry earrings and platform shoes; my bridesmaids in Liberty florals and turbans fastened with pink cloth roses, wearing fake eyelashes, cheeks painted with little red clown circles; and Andrew's bearded artist friends from Leeds in jeans. Then, arriving from London in huge American cars, came a long Greek procession of men in shiny mohair suits and little old ladies in black. Andrew was so worried about my father's reaction that he'd had stomach pains for three weeks and had been to see a doctor, who told him to relax and eat boiled fish. But Daddy knew when he'd lost and behaved quite graciously, at the ceremony and at home, where we had a lovely wedding breakfast in the garden. But again the difference between my family's worldview and mine seemed pointed, and what I saw as a languid afternoon of drinking champagne under the trees looked, to my parents, like a circus. When I phoned from the airport to say goodbye, my mother exclaimed, "Darling! What am I going to do? There are bearded people still in the vegetable garden, and I think they're smoking marijuana!" Little did she know that, a few hours earlier, her new son-in-law had been one of them. He got stoned in an upstairs bathroom, and I had to send a search party to bring him down for his speech, in which he cheekily thanked my father for all he had done in bringing us together!

Our honeymoon was my first time in Greece, and turned out to be an adventure with small creatures. We'd feast at seaside grills where the "menu" was a display of fish that had been swimming an hour earlier. (I got ill from overindulging on whitebait and retsina.) A friend at work, Georgina Russell (now Lady Boothby), had offered the use of her family's home on the isle of Spetse. (We had to ignore the friendly mice who lived in the rafters.) Other friends had a warren of rabbits in the backyard, and I was asked to choose my favorite: It was cooked for my dinner. But Greece started to get into my blood, as it was in Andrew's, and we were to return every year, never exhausting its islands, its history, and its hospitality.

My new in-laws had moved to Eastbourne, a seaside resort town on the south coast of England, where to supplement his income Andrew had bought a restaurant that his father would manage, so we took over their apartment in London. Andrew was still lecturing in Leeds but worked at the restaurant on weekends. So my early married life was circumscribed by a geographical triangle: Andrew would leave Leeds on Thursday night, drive 200 miles to London, then pick me up Friday afternoon after work and drive the 80 miles to Eastbourne for the weekend, dropping me off in London on Sunday night and continuing to Leeds again early Monday morning. This insane schedule was to last for ten years.

My salary of 900 pounds a year—less than $2,000—didn't begin to cover the kind of clothes I was expected to wear. None of the editors were paid extravagantly, but sometimes they got designer discounts, and sometimes they just bought clothes instead of food. I had to make most of my own. I'd go to Theatreland Fabrics near Soho Square, run by an Indian man who supplied material for the saris worn by his countrywomen living in London, as well as for the costumes of all the chorus lines of the Shaftesbury Avenue theaters. I earned extra cash by sewing broken zippers back into pants for colleagues (at one pound each). Sometimes I was given shoes from the fashion closet that were no longer needed—green wedge platforms and blue ankle-strap sandals and shiny yellow boots—and I'd plan my color scheme from the feet up. For shirts, which are awfully complicated to make, I'd shop in bargain basements and vintage clothing shops. I did my best, but it was difficult to keep my wardrobe up to the fashion department's exacting and mercurial standards. One day I was steered into a corner by Grace's new assistant, Patricia McRoberts, an heiress to the Shell Oil fortune, who drove a Ferrari *and* a Maserati. "Look," she whispered, "I know you don't earn any money, but you really do have to dress better." I was deeply humiliated, but I'm a resolute person and I thought: I will try harder, even if I have to fight every inch of the fucking way.

FASHION AT THE beginning of the 1970s was psychedelically colored, whimsically decorative, influenced by the flower-child culture. The pages of *Vogue* had a dreamy innocence punctuated by the odd, startling shot of eccentricity, such as a model's hair turned into a bird's nest, or extraordinary, Kabuki-painted faces. We were promoting the fantasies of the wonderful crop of recent graduates from the Royal College of Art—the ethereal screened prints of Zandra Rhodes, the ethnic layers of Bill Gibb, the op-art textiles of Ossie Clark—while also discovering the new consciousness of fashion in more accessible, wearable chic with a sense of downmarket, throwaway elegance. Vivienne Westwood pushed the envelope of street style pioneered by Mary Quant, launching a succession of King's Road boutiques with increasingly edgy names: Let It Rock; Too Fast to Live, Too Young to Die; Sex; and later, Seditionaries and World's End.

Since this was, after all, British *Vogue*, and since England had had a glorious moment in the 1960s when the rest of the world turned to us to observe the bright young things of fashion, we were still expected to reflect some jingoistic pride. But *Vogue* still went around the globe for the photos. There were epic trips to Egypt, Israel, Sri Lanka, Machu Picchu. On a trip to the Soviet Union with Jerry Hall modeling, the Kremlin insisted that the film be developed before leaving the country, but Norman Parkinson kept the best rolls of each shot and smuggled them out in case the Russian version of Fotomat screwed up.

I heard such stories secondhand—assistants never got to go anywhere. I spent my days sweating in a summertime studio (then and now, the British don't put much stock in air conditioning) or freezing my butt off in a wintry park—it wasn't glamorous, but it was the best possible grounding: Fashion Skills 101. A good editor has to be a sponge, absorbing other people's style, looking for the intricacies that occur on the runway and on the street. It's a constant conversation and observation. (To this moment, I can tell you what everybody in the office was wearing last week or my friends had on at the restaurant last night.) We put it all into the computer in our heads, download it and reuse it, adapting the rules of taste that get broken and remade a bit each season. But we're not starting from ground zero. When I make apple crumble, I'm always adjusting the recipe, and we do that with clothes. (Everybody does it. Editors just do it professionally.) One season it's narrow pants; the next, wide; the third, either way but with high heels rather than plat-forms—a transmutating, metamorphosing, cross-fertilizing process. And once we've been emboldened, there's no turning back.

Watching Sheila Wetton at a sitting was a revelation, especially if the clothes were familiar or mundane, as inevitably p-and-s was.

She sometimes let me choose the accessories, and if she didn't approve, she would quietly take off the offending item until I got it right—adding a green bangle to the orange jacket because it made the jacket jump, or knowing that an Arran sweater with khaki pants would be sharpened with the collar of a white shirt peeking out. Sheila taught me not to be afraid of putting the same colors together—that a spectrum of beiges or grays could have more impact than a rainbow. She'd contemplate the seemingly imponderable question of how to do yet another sweater set, or spend hours tying and retying scarves until she found the exact hue, print, and drape to renew the look. Then again, sometimes she would say, "Make it blurred, make it quick, I have to get home for lunch."

David Bailey and his sittings were always an event, "Bails" being the prototype for the louche character in the 1966 Antonioni movie *Blow-Up*. We'd get a model ready in the dressing rooms, perfectly coordinated with coat, dress, stockings, hat, jewelry, and gloves. The studio door would close. We'd wait outside for an hour, and the girl would come out completely unwrapped except for the coat. He always wanted the sexy picture (and often the girl herself), and the fashion editor always wanted to showcase the clothes. It was a constant tussle, and he could reduce an adversary to tears by putting a dead mouse in her hotel room or rat droppings in her bed—different stunts for different people, depending on what he thought they needed. But he knew how to make a woman look vulnerable and provocative, was a master at lighting, and understood every aspect of a model's face and hair and body. The pictures were always gorgeous.

Sometimes we'd shoot in Bailey's North London playboy pad, which was painted all black and adorned with exotic plants and pet parrots, which were allowed to fly about the dressing room and shit everywhere. My first task when we worked there was to cover everything in the room with sheets of plastic. But I got my revenge. One of the birds choked on the top of a ballpoint pen I'd left lying about after a sitting, fell into the toilet, and drowned. Bailey didn't speak to me for months.

By the winter of 1971, the British economy was in big trouble, and the consequences were becoming shockingly obvious in daily life. Striking workers picketed, power was rationed, a three-day week was enforced, and we had to leave the office before four o'clock, when the lights went out. There was an incongruous, quaint glow of candlelight coming from office buildings all over the city, a not unpleasant effect, but there were IRA bombings too. Once when I was going home on a double-decker bus, the regular route out of central London was closed off after a bomb threat at Selfridges, the department store in Oxford Street, and the driver was too flustered to find an alternative route. I sat behind him directing the bus on a circuitous path through Regent's Park.

I was in a slump too. Assiduous effort did not seem to translate to promotion—a "good name" was a better career enhancer. When Emma Soames, a granddaughter of Winston Churchill, was added to the masthead (the list of staff names in the front of the magazine), I was consumed with jealousy—she was a perfectly good editor, but she was younger than I and had worked there for a shorter time. I was determined to make myself noticed despite my lack of pedigree, and I hit upon an idea to cover the Paris ready-to-wear. Andrew and I ferried across the English Channel from Dover to Calais in our green Porsche and drove to Paris, where we found a dumpy hotel near the Place du Trocadéro. Our first morning, anticipating a romantic breakfast in bed, I found my croissant garnished with a cockroach. I literally threw my tray up to the ceiling, and am sure my scream was heard across the Seine! Entrance to the shows at the designers' salons was restricted to senior editors and controlled by security gestapo, so I figured I would get in literally through the back door. I went to the trade exhibitions at the Port de Versailles, where the retailers place their orders. I prepared a report with dozens of sketches on new labels like Thierry Mugler and French Connection and presented my notebook to Miss Miller when I returned.

My scheme worked: The following year, I was included as part of the team sent to Paris. Although I was pleased with my clever strategizing, I was developing a reputation for being pushy and aggressive. (It was all a charade: I was still racked with such self-doubt that I often left the house crying in the morning.) A junior editor took me aside one day and said, "Do you realize how much everybody hates you?" I was stunned—little old me? But it didn't dampen my ambition for one moment. I was going to be accepted.

Determination finally earned me more responsibility. I was assigned to research the lingerie market, where I frequently crossed paths with the lingerie editor for *Harpers & Queen*, a fashionable society magazine rather like *Town and Country*. Her name was Anna Wintour, and we quickly recognized each other as fellow foot soldiers of fashion (although she was always better dressed than I was), sitting together at tedious industry lunches and meeting up at showrooms to peruse racks of Maidenform bras and flannel robes, two ambitious neophytes glad to have each other's company and conversation. Without a crystal ball, there would have been no way of predicting our future journey of crossed and parallel paths. She was serious but not humorless, determined but not devious, obviously as frustrated as I was at the limitations of our current bailiwick: You can do only so much with lingerie, and we weren't even doing the creative part, just researching the market and reporting back to more senior people.

At the same time, I was put in charge of the smallest *Vogue* sittings. I was so proud of my first shoot that I stuck the photograph—a jumbled neckful of chains, chokers, baubles, and beads—on my locker door. It was a talented South African photographer named Barry Lategan who guided me through my baby steps as an editor. Barry had done many of the innovative covers that made me gasp and had been kind enough to take my wedding pictures. He taught me about studio manners: when to shut up, when to chatter, how to avoid violating the tacit hierarchy of who reports to whom. I learned to arrive early, put the music on *loud*, chat with the makeup artist about star signs, make sure the hairdresser had a plug for his curling tongs and the model had her glass of wine and the photographer felt he was the best thing since Cecil Beaton. There's a subtle psychological side to a sitting, and a good editor learns to prop up fragile egos, finesse power struggles, and smooth ruffled feathers. Once I even saved Barry. He had just put on some music, but after I heard two bars I ran over and ripped the record off with a screech. It was George Harrison, and the model that day was Patti Boyd, who had just left her Beatle for Eric Clapton. We averted disaster by seconds.

But I was still not on the masthead, being considered too junior (and, I suspected, not posh enough). I then learned a very sound lesson in career negotiations: that other options provide invaluable leverage. Suzy Menkes, who was covering fashion for the London *Evening Standard*, had made one of those vague, offhand remarks like, "If you ever want to come and work for me . . ." But I had a real offer to be the assistant to Michael Roberts, then fashion editor for the London *Sunday Times*, whose editor-in-chief was Harold Evans (not yet married to Tina Brown, who was forging her own brilliant career at *Tatler*). When I went to be interviewed, Evans produced several photographs and asked, "Which one would you use?" I chose wrong: I picked the full-length picture that showed the clothes, and he liked the sexy picture. But the job was mine if I wanted it, a lateral move, with no increase in pay.

It was a big moment when I told Grace that I had another job offer. She didn't react in any of the ways I could have predicted. Instead, she pushed me into the fashion closet and shut the door. "Look," she said fiercely, "fashion is all about working with color. These are *newspapers*. What are you going to do with four hundred words and two black-and-white photographs a week?" But I'd made my point. Both Grace and Sheila recognized that I had fashion instincts, which had nothing to do with the way I dressed myself. It had to do with a feeling, an eye, a penchant for the ever-changing world of clothes. In February 1974, my name went on the masthead under the general heading of "Fashion," and I was put in charge of the budget pages, called "More Dash Than Cash." Everything the model wore had to add up to less than 60 pounds, about $100, which was exactly the way I dressed myself—and was certainly why I got the assignment. I thought that affordable fashion on a shoestring was an important theme for a lot of readers, given the state of the economy, and I tackled the task of finding those clothes with all the seriousness and energy I'd seen applied to the heady excesses of couture. I'd get khakis from army surplus stores, belts from Woolworth's, tights from Boots the Chemists. Once while I was choosing clothes in the management offices of a well-known High Street store, a closet door opened and out tumbled all the Gucci handbags they were knocking off. As I mastered the art of dressing on a dime, I was given bigger sittings, better clothes, the best models.

My husband was always boasting to his friends about his close proximity to models, a kind of gilt by association. One day I dealt with that. With a lot of preparatory fanfare, I invited home a lovely model named Susan Moncur, and Andrew made sure our living room was filled with an appropriate reception committee of wide-eyed, expectant men. Susan walked in wearing a ragged sweater, no makeup, and a pair of bent eyeglasses held together with tape, as ordinary-looking as I knew she would be. A photograph in a magazine is a chimerical construction, having little to do with real life. Off the pages and in their natural habitat, models rarely look like the painted images of fashion spreads. The men mumbled a few words of hello and wandered off to the pub to drown their disappointment. I never heard any model lust in our home again.

# 6

THERE'S A RHYTHM to the life of a fashion magazine. The editors
are assembling a group of ideas that will tell the reader where she's
going next season with her clothes, and the ready-to-wear shows
provide the raw material. During my early days in the business,
shows were not the theatrical extravaganzas they are now, but rather
homey little affairs, with runway models who were not household
names. There were no flashing strobe lights, no CNN, no Elton
John, Madonna, or Courtney Love in the front row, no shouts of
"Linda! Christy! Claudia!" and no grand proclamations that
"Brown is the new black"—just an insular group of editors looking
for inspiration, hoping to find one outfit from a collection that
could make the transition from show to sitting, from theory to
practice.

Once the clothes were in our mind's eye, ideas for photographing
them were gleaned from office brainstorming or from history or
pop culture or street life—say, the Renaissance, or Stonehenge, or
*Play It Again, Sam*, or "Send In the Clowns," or motorcycles, or
gypsies. Sometimes we were rather precious: Stories headlined

"Tutu Divine" or "Oh, What's the Matador?" would elicit derisive guffaws in today's more sophisticated climate. (One editor ingeniously came up with the title "Cream It," a rude British term for masturbation. We decided she didn't have much experience.) When I had established the concept of the sitting, its approximate look and feel, I'd call in clothes from the shows that fit my theme, put them on a rolling rack and wheel them into Miss Miller's office. I always arranged them according to color, each outfit accessorized and assembled from hat to shoes.

Miss Miller's office was calm and orderly, with a Standard typewriter, a 35-millimeter projector for viewing slides, and a blackout blind on the window. One wall was covered in emerald green felt, pinned ad hoc with a few photographs: Lord Snowdon in a stone fountain shaped like a lotus flower; Paul McCartney's daughter Stella as a baby, twenty-five years before she was named the designer for Chloé. A metal dress rail was installed on the length of the back wall for the final selection of clothes to be photographed, and I would have rehearsed my pitch to Miss Miller—I really had to *sell* the story to her. (Years later, Grace Coddington would say I became so self-confident that I'd come out of her office with an approved lot of white dresses and return from the sitting having photographed nothing but black.)

Most of the time, I worked in the studios or in various locations around town. One story was shot in the ladies' room of Harrods—which was complicated because people kept coming in to use it. Another time we were photographing the child star Tatum O'Neal in the London streets, right before she won the Academy Award for *Paper Moon*, and a truck driver who was parked in our way refused to move.

"Do you want me to punch him in the mouth?" asked Tatum's father, Ryan, cordially.

"No, that's all right," I said hastily, "we'll find another way." The stage mother of another young actress who was modeling for us was having an affair with her daughter's bodyguard, which we had to pretend not to notice. But we did have fun on a shoot with some famous male sports stars who got very ... excited carrying the models on their shoulders!

After each sitting, I would be back in Miss Miller's office, the blackout shade drawn, as the photos taken under my aegis were projected onto the wall, and I waited to hear if the work had pleased or not. The latter was a dreaded contingency. Once I discovered too late that we should never show a girl in a skirt walking together with a girl in pants, that Miss Miller thought this was "dykey." (You only find out about some rules after you've broken them.) Sheila Wetton had to supervise all my sittings for a while after that to make sure I didn't do anything else stupid. But we were allowed to be pretty risqué—it was no problem showing naked breasts in a lingerie story, or any other story, for that matter. The British are not as puritanical about nudity as Americans: The American model Barbara Neuman once asked me to write to her mother explaining, "It was in the spirit of the trip that Barbara's nipples show in these photographs."

When the pictures were chosen, they were laid out by the art director, and then the fight for pages would begin, with each editor competing for the limited space available in each issue. The habits of professional photographers vary considerably: Some work in a spare, minimalist way, shooting little footage, and some take a hundred shots of every outfit, most of which will never see the light of day. Models are paid for their time (actually very demo-cratically—when they work for magazines, the superstars get the same as unknowns), but photographers are paid only when their work makes it into the pages, unless they are under contract. It's depressing when so much goes for naught, but that's the reality of the business. Often I was dissatisfied with the final selection and thought the page should have a bubble coming out of the model's mouth, the way dialogue is printed in comic strips, saying, "Liz didn't like this layout. There were *much* better pictures."

Because of the hours spent together on location in faraway places, the lives and loves of editors, photographers, models, hair-dressers, and makeup artists become endlessly, sometimes dis-astrously, intertwined. Just as movie sets are notorious dens of iniquity, with steamy relationships between costars replicating the ones between characters, the professional alliances in the world of fashion sometimes tumble into the personal. The hazard is self-evident: There's a subtext of sexual energy to many shoots—it's right there in the pictures. Sex sells. It jumps off the page and demands attention. The players in these scenarios are often attractive and uninhibited, and it's tempting and convenient to have the location equivalent of an office romance. As in the movie business, there's also a certain casting-couch element to the fashion world. I've been at sittings where two models fought over the last outfit, knowing that whoever left the set with the photographer would end up in his bed, possibly enhancing her career.

Sometimes the game turned into musical chairs. Marie Helvin, an exotic Hawaiian model, married David Bailey, replacing Penelope Tree. Bailey had also had a relationship with Jean Shrimpton and been married to Catherine Deneuve. We lost track of all the women Bailey romanced, although he's now married to the delightful former model Catherine Dyer, with a passel of children, which he swore he'd never have. Shrimpton's younger sister Chrissie was at one time the girlfriend of Mick Jagger, and Jerry Hall was the girlfriend of Bryan Ferry, the lead singer of Roxy Music. Then there was a sighting of Mick and Jerry: Everybody change partners and dance.

If you didn't want to play at the game of recreational sex, you had to make that clear. The first time I met the photographer Alex Chatelain, after a Kenzo show in Paris, he took me to the Brasserie Lorraine and ordered a seduction meal—two dozen royale oysters washed down with Sancerre—thinking he was going to get me drunk. But Alex didn't know about my hollow leg (or about Andrew's training in martial arts). I drank him under the table. At the end of the evening, I walked *him* up the Champs Élysées, where he had to stop and pee in the bushes, and shoved him in the door of his apartment. Then I walked myself back to my hotel singing "La Vie en Rose." That was the beginning of a lovely—platonic— friendship, although I did get to see his penis, as did everyone else on a shoot in Scotland, when Alex pulled down his pants and flashed us. That little prank earned him the name "Arctic Whale" because what he was flashing looked so cold and white.

Things didn't always turn out so well. I'd become friends with Donna Jordan, a feisty, fast-talking blonde I met on my first solo visit to New York for the opening of the Fiorucci boutique in 1974. She'd been part of Andy Warhol's Factory and introduced me to the flea markets of the city, always a great resource for sittings. Donna fell in love with a photographer named Oliviero Toscani, who later shot and art directed the notorious Benetton advertising campaigns showing parents hunched over a dying child and babies with bloody umbilical cords. Then, fatefully, I booked a rangy model named Kirsti Moseng for a shoot with Oliviero, and the two of *them* fell in love at first sight. One dreadful evening, Andrew and I went out to dinner with Oliviero and Donna at Michael Caine's restaurant called Langan's Brasserie, near Piccadilly Circus. Oliviero made some excuse to leave early and went to see Kirsti. Donna didn't know yet, but I did. I love gossip as much as anyone, but it can be rather stressful to be privy to information that you know would be devastating to a friend. These days if someone asks, "Want to know a secret?" I'm almost inclined to say, "I'd rather not." But it was the real thing between Toscani and Kirsti: They've been together ever since. Donna married the late Andrea Ballo, and their extremely glamorous daughter, Kate Ballo, was photographed for the September 1997 *Harper's Bazaar*.

During those high times, there were a lot of illegal highs available. At a sitting in an elegant apartment across from Regent's Park, I opened the refrigerator to store the film, and out fell a bottle of amyl nitrate, unmistakable for its rotten-egg smell. In the late 1970s we booked the sultry American model Gia Carangi to pose in an Adrian Cartmel black chiffon dress on Salvador Dali's famous red lip-shaped sofa that we had shipped to our studio. I had no idea of her relationship with drugs at the time and couldn't understand her confused and spacey manner. When she started crying in the middle of the sitting, we had to bring in another girl. (Gia eventually died of drug-related AIDS in 1986.) One famous French model who arrived at a sitting with a white cocaine mustache was incapable of standing up, and had to be sent home. But most people were secretive about their drug habits—I'd walk into a studio bathroom at an inauspicious moment to see lines of cocaine on the counter. A model's boyfriend would show up at a sitting, and they'd disappear into the bathroom, either to get high or get laid. Generally the sex took slightly longer.

I was terrifically impressed by some of the boyfriends—I swooned like a teenager when a model called Tara Shannon showed up with a member of the Average White Band—but not by the drugs. I did go to see *Star Wars* after smoking a couple of joints—quite a trip—but chemicals never really attracted me. It was more about booze with my crowd, and we never thought that getting sloshed on beer was risky business. For a story in British *Vogue* about the wardrobes of its own editors, I was photographed in a tweed coat and quoted as saying, "It is essential to look healthy even when hungover."

My insurance policy for a great sitting was getting everybody nicely plastered and relaxed. Once we took Clio Goldsmith, niece of the late outspoken billionaire Sir James Goldsmith, to a chateau in Épernay, the champagne region of France, for an "advertorial": Fashion editors were sometimes hired by manufacturers and retailers to style their advertising pages with a more editorial point of view. In those days, advertising imagery lagged at least six months behind the look of the magazine fashion pages and the clients hoped that the editorial perspective would ensure the newest and most sophisticated photography. From the opening shot, we were plied with the hometown beverage. Even the food was cooked in champagne. We were soon so drunk that we had a lunchtime cream fight on the lawn and poured a bucket of water over the client's girlfriend, who was being photographed out of politeness to the client. It was very bad behavior—a bit like boarding school—and such fun.

Sometimes the fun went too far. I went to the Caribbean island Bequia with Alex Chatelain to shoot romantic pirate looks on a girl and boy seemingly washed up on a desert island. One night after dinner, we got rowdy playing strip Ping-Pong and everybody ran into the sea, kneeling down in the surf to cover up the nudity of a losing game. A guest at the hotel thought we were standing, and she dove off the dock head first into two feet of water, breaking her back. There was no way to expedite emergency medical attention on a remote island, and during a seemingly interminable wait for aid, somebody in our crew fed her Quaaludes, after which I started thinking about packing them in a travel kit along with my toothbrush. Alex saw her some time later, fully recovered after spending an entire year in hospital.

In 1976 British *Vogue* celebrated its sixtieth anniversary with a Diamond Jubilee issue. One sitting involved a diamond photographed on the model's tongue, shot in such close-up that all you saw was a huge rock on a pink slope. The security guard assigned to protect the jewel was a wreck: If the model swallowed, choked, or inhaled, she would have to be placed under house arrest until nature took its course.

By 1979, I was starting to get some plum assignments and was among the first fashion journalists allowed into Beijing, still called Peking in the West. We traveled on Ethiopian Airlines, which provided free tickets as long as we put a picture of their plane in the magazine. (On limited budgets, we made strange bargains with the devil.) We flew twenty-six hours, via Addis Ababa and Bombay, suspending all normal standards of comfort and hygiene. China smelled of garlic and mothballs. We stayed in a huge hotel of faded imperial glory, where everything was covered in layers of dust, and a female custodian on each floor stood sentinel in the corridor outside the rooms. Grace Coddington was to shoot the editorial pages, and I was to do advertorials for a shop called Regine. Both of us wanted to use the glorious graphic image of the Great Wall as a backdrop, but I won. I was rather like a Rottweiler about it, and I did have the shop owner, who was funding some of the trip, on my side. A group of Chinese athletes who happened to be running along the wall were delighted to make our model, Kim Charleton, an impromptu teammate for the camera.

Everywhere we went, we had to explain what credit cards were, and everywhere we photographed, a crowd of hundreds would gather to look at the strangers, like the Munchkins checking out Dorothy. We'd brought Polaroid cameras as gifts for our guides and local dignitaries (and sent film as Christmas presents for years afterward). At one of the many formal and multicourse banquets, a dish was put before us that our guide told us was dog. Such a menu sounded all too probable—we'd passed restaurants where we saw dogs and cats tied up outside the kitchen door—and we discreetly pushed it aside, not wanting to offend by acting revolted at native custom. But the guide laughed and said it was really sea cucumber. I ate it, only later realizing that I'd eaten a sea slug. In Datong, where we were jolted by an earthquake, the model Esme announced that she had to return to the United States for the opening of her producer boyfriend's musical. The nearest airport was probably 2,000 miles away, so she wasn't going anywhere, but we had to calm her down. For a while, it seemed that *none* of us was getting home: Our Ethiopian plane, missing a part, was delayed past the time our visas had expired. For twenty-four hours we were confined to cots in the Beijing airport compound, playing gin rummy and wondering if we'd be starting Pekingese *Vogue*.

THE END OF the 1970s was a watershed for fashion, with a sharp and revolutionary turn toward the United States. It was the American cultural landscape—its music, films, nightlife, and designers—that seemed to offer the most exciting and inspirational ideas, and British *Vogue* was pulled out of its long epoch of European fantasy. Little was happening in English fashion, besides the launch of Katharine Hamnett, who made the headlines with political slogan T-shirts, and of the team of Elizabeth and David Emmanuel, who became famous for designing the ruffly wedding dress of Lady Diana Spencer. A few Italians were catching our interest, such as Romeo Gigli with his sensuous, body-skimming designs, and as always we paid attention to the French. But America was the delightful new kid on the block. Grace Coddington went to New York and came home to announce, "This is *it*—how modern

96

women should dress." Sportswear entered our consciousness: the minimalistic pants and wrap dresses of Calvin Klein; the outdoorsy vision of Ralph Lauren, with its underlying worship of all things British. We threw out everything else in our closets.

Just as the nexus of designers shifted to America, so did our perceptions of the feminine ideal. Replacing the Pre-Raphaelite was a robust, athletic American girl-next-door, the avatars being Christie Brinkley, Kelly Emberg, and the Dickinson sisters, Janice and Debbie. The new paradigm of female beauty had arrived by way of Iowa, looking as if she had only recently relinquished her prom-queen crown and could bench-press her body weight. Fitness was the new mantra. Grace got me included in the group British *Vogue* sent to the New York collections in 1980, not least, I suspect, because she wanted a jogging partner, although *that* phase lasted about a minute. The doormen at the fabled Algonquin Hotel were quite amused at the sight of two purported style mavens in blue tracksuits, puffing through the lobby and collapsing into the chairs once occupied by Dorothy Parker, Robert Benchley, and their circle.

There was a certain amount of squabbling and competition about which editor got to shoot which outfits, but Grace and I managed to be the best of rivals and the best of friends, our office affinity gradually spilling into the social. I think it worked because we matched each other in our limitless devotion to fashion; each of us could discuss any detail microscopically. I was opinionated and self-confident, but Grace was one of the few people whose judgment I respected. She was unlike most women at *Vogue* who had grown up in stately homes, and when I learned that her mother had given her a ham sandwich for dinner every night of her childhood, I stopped being so intimidated.

My only serious problem at work was that I felt I deserved a more senior title than fashion editor: I wanted to be second in command to Grace, who was fashion director. Grace was my superior, overseeing my independent work as a fashion editor but occasionally relying on my collaboration for her sittings. I loved working with her, but I wanted recognition for my role.

97

The great thing about Grace and I working together was that we never argued, except over one thing: My only quarrel with her, then and now, is that she is pathologically late, and I constantly had to lie, telling her that an appointment was an hour earlier than actually scheduled. One morning while we were working at the New York collections, she kept me waiting for so long in the hotel lobby that I exploded.

"How can you be so inconsiderate?" I screamed. "Now everyone at the sitting will be delayed, and it's just plain rude."

All camaraderie and friendship drained out of her face, her body visibly stiffened, and the rest of the day was spent in stony silence, except for a necessary snarl of commands. By the afternoon, Beatrix Miller had been told of my insubordination, and she asked me to join her in a cab to the next show. I didn't know if I'd be fired, if my career was screeching to a premature end on the streets of New York. She was kind in her reprimand. "Liz," she began, "you've got to calm down." Since I've become a manager myself, I understand that it's rarely productive to lose control in a fit of pique, and I also know that there are late people and punctual people, that the latter are prompt despite weather or traffic or acts of God. Most of the time, I try to set an example of promptness as good sportsmanship. And when I want to have lunch with Grace at one o'clock, I still tell her noon.

I WAS HITTING my professional stride as a fashion editor when I started working with the photographer Bruce Weber in 1980. Bruce's forte is the expansive, pastoral location shoot. It involves a cast of dozens, a journey, a narrative, an emotional intensity that wraps us up for days. For our first trip together, we went to the Greek island of Skíathos and then the Halkadiki Peninsula, two places I'd never visited despite the annual excursions Andrew and I made to the land of his heritage. The beach is always a good studio, with vast expanses of light and sky, and the clothes were informal and spontaneous—swimsuit bottoms with sweatshirt tops, terrycloth robes and suede shorts—pricey but unstudied.

The shoot had such a freewheeling atmosphere that the line between work and play got blurred. The proprietor of the boat shop handed me a bill for the waterskiing equipment we'd used, and I nearly fainted—Miss Miller would have had my head on a platter. And this was long before a marina on a remote Greek island would accept Visa. In desperation I turned to Chris Lawrence, the travel agent and a good friend who'd organized the trip and accompanied us. He didn't seem at all perturbed. "So we won't pay," Chris said. And we actually fled like thieves. In order to get away earlier than scheduled, we employed the services of another minor felon in our group who knew how to steal the little stickers that go on airline tickets to change a flight, a malfeasance that bumped other people off the plane. To this day, for all I know, I may be a fugitive from justice in Skíathos.

Bruce was always discovering new models, in coffee shops, on the street, on the beach. The girls were unadorned, freckled, bespectacled, with unplucked brows and just-out-of-bed hair. After the highly processed, cosmeticized looks of the past decade, he was creating a new standard of beauty that had never been recognized before. And there were *always* great-looking guys around Bruce, even though Bea Miller and Grace Coddington were telling us, "*Please*, there are too many boys in the pictures—nobody will see the clothes." Sometimes they were unknowns whom we seemed to acquire like the Pied Piper, waiters and lifeguards and motel clerks—Bruce once called me right before a trip and said, "The pool cleaner is coming. He's gorgeous." Some were (or were soon to become) well known, at least for their ego and attitude. Matt Dillon was annoyed that one Los Angeles sitting wasn't just about *him*. "My agent didn't tell me I had to be with all these models," he complained.

"Pinch a bottom from time to time," I said, "and you'll feel better."

We were shooting in Los Angeles during a terrible hurricane—Queen Elizabeth happened to be in town at the same time, and the papers were full of apologies for hurricaning all over the royal visitors. The grassy outdoor carpeting of the Bel-Air Hotel was sodden, and we were all a bit bummed out by the less-than-dependably-perfect California weather. But the skies cleared for a day of shooting by the pool at the grand home of the producer Robert Evans. An aspiring actor named Kevin Costner was the model who'd been booked that day, but he became petulant and lethargic. When he asked for the four hundredth time how much longer it would take, I said, "We're fine now; you can go," and finished the sitting with somebody else. I found out too late that a houseguest named Richard Gere had been lounging around the kitchen.

The best fashion photography springs from the heart and the memory as much as it does from the runway. Bruce Weber's photos were always about *something*, and they were always emotional. Our most meaningful sitting together was in Nebraska in 1981. Bruce had wanted to shoot the roadside diners of Kansas, like a post-modern Edward Hopper series, but I'd been spellbound by the poetry and visual imagery of the Willa Cather novels Bruce had given me to read and persuaded him to move the location to Red Cloud, where Cather grew up in the late nineteenth century. After many long phone conversations with Bruce, I pulled together trunks of antique clothing, blanket coats from Ralph Lauren, plaid skirts from Perry Ellis, smocks from Laura Ashley, Aquascutum tweeds, laced boots from Manolo Blahnik, and Edwardian children's clothes. We took over the whole township—the schoolhouse, the cornfields, the pig farms. The model Tracy Fitzpatrick turned her tanned face and blue eyes up to the wide skies and perfectly incarnated Cather's words: "Her complexion is firm with an outdoor wholesomeness. The red in her cheeks is the red that comes from the bite of the wind."

There was a lot of tenderness in those pictures. It was a kind of completion for me too, a Janus look backward and forward. I'd put a tiny Manx brooch at the throat of Tracy's shirt in one of the pictures, a little nod to the pioneering women of my own ancestry. But this was also the moment when I could finally see my way clearly into the future. For the past five years, there had been a terrible shadow across my personal life: I'd been unable to get pregnant and failed to conceive after repeated bouts of fertility treatment. Finally Andrew and I were in the last weeks of adoption proceedings, and our first little boy was on his way to us. After years of struggle, I knew that I was going to be a mother.

# 7

I HESITATE TO write this—I know it sounds illogical and unlikely—but the trajectory of my ordeal with infertility and ultimately cancer began with a yeast infection.

My generation ushered in the sexual revolution, but it wasn't so revolutionary for me. I had exactly two sexual partners before Andrew and I met and mated for life, like swans. But somehow during my extremely non-swinging single days, I got PID—pelvic inflammatory disease. I didn't know it at the time. I only knew I had a yeast infection, called thrush in Britain. Nothing worrisome—it was practically a rite of passage for women, and still is, if the television commercials for home remedies are any indication, but in those days I went to a clinic, where I was given yellow pessaries to deal with the itch. Yeast can mask other, more ominous kinds of sexually transmitted infections, and you don't have to be promiscuous to get one—just unlucky. Without warning, I developed a vaginal infection that spread to my fallopian tubes and became salpingitis, a PID that ultimately made me infertile.

I was oblivious to any such problem until ten years later, when

Andrew and I were married and trying in vain to get pregnant, although I should have been clued in because we'd been having unprotected sex for quite some time. I'd tried the Pill for about six months, but it made me completely frigid, like the Victorian ladies who'd lie back and think of England. So we were just … careful, which is, of course, exactly how so many women get pregnant. I'd gone for checkups on the sort of haphazard, cavalier basis as most presumably healthy young women: Every few years, I'd been examined by a GP with the National Health Service. This time when I told my doctor that I was failing to conceive, he assured me there was absolutely nothing wrong with me except that I was working too hard. He sent me home with a chart to monitor my ovulation, and for one solid year, I took my temperature every morning, the moment I woke up, before eating or drinking anything. When the mercury in the thermometer moved two dots, from 98.6 to 98.8, that meant I was about to ovulate and had three days of deliberate, baby-making sex—the reverse of the rhythm method. Andrew still refers to this as the best time of our marriage.

He was not so pleased with the next phase: semen analyses and sperm counts. For reasons involving earlier girlfriends, he was pretty sure he was capable of getting the job done, but he still had to undergo tests with such charming names as "bovine mucus" and "hamster egg penetration." (The former determines the swimming skills of a man's sperm, the latter their ability to fertilize a human egg.) Being told his equipment was in fine working order was scarcely compensation for the mortifying task of "producing samples" in a hospital toilet stall and waiting to be told whether he was man enough to knock up his wife.

There's a lot of folkloric advice about getting pregnant: licorice, sesame seeds, raspberry tea, enough garlic to ward off vampires— I heard and tried it all. People suggested psychics and astrologers, chants and incantations, all manner of food and drink. I'd consult the horoscope columns, abandoning my usual skepticism about the metaphysical and the intangible. And I got crazily superstitious, playing mind games on myself: I'd be crossing the road and think: *If the light doesn't change before I reach the curb, then I'm pregnant.* I'd recite the school rhyme every English child knows about magpies, the black and white birds that are as common in the U.K. as pigeons in New York: "One for sorrow, two for joy, three for a girl, four for a boy, five for silver, six for gold, seven for a secret never to be told." If I saw four magpies foraging in the field, I'd think: *Maybe I'll have a son.*

But nothing was happening. One of my colleagues suggested that I visit a private gynecologist in London's Harley Street, which was and still is to the world of medicine what Wall Street is to finance and Madison Avenue to advertising. She prescribed something called a fertility "booster," which I now realize must have been Clomid. I reveal my ignorance with some chagrin, because women today are such well-informed consumers of their own health care (a perspective we endorse and foster in *Bazaar*); at the time, it didn't occur to me to question the doctor's authority, to ask: Are these hormones? Vitamins? Muscle relaxers? Stimulants? I just took them.

After three months, the doctor felt it was foolish to waste any more time, that we should find out why a perfectly normal and fit thirty-two-year-old woman wasn't getting pregnant, and she suggested I see a friend of hers, Professor Ian Craft at the Royal Free Hospital in Hampstead, a leafy part of North London. ("Professor" is an honorific granted to British physicians of a certain stature.) Craft was a distinguished-looking middle-aged man with thick graying hair who talked at the speed of light, rather gruff and no-nonsense but still avuncular and kind. I don't particularly want or need a charming bedside manner—I'd prefer to have doctors shoot straight rather than sugar-coat. Craft said I would need a surgical procedure called laparoscopy to determine what was wrong: While I was under general anesthesia, he would make a small incision near my navel and insert a long, thin fiberoptic telescope to look around.

I was groggy but awake, my abdomen bruised and tender, when Professor Craft came into my room after the surgery and announced: "There is no way in your current condition you're going to have children." Both of my fallopian tubes were completely blocked from the salpingitis. Each tube is only a few milli-meters in diameter—about the size of a hair—and bacteria from an infection makes it sticky; the inner walls of that narrow tube literally stick together and ultimately scar over. The end of the tube normally looks like a tiny hand, but when it's infected it balloons out so that it looks like a golf club—this is actually called clubbing. It's quite common for women who've had PID to end up with a tubal pregnancy, because the fertilized egg gets stuck in the sticky fallopian tube and fails to proceed to the uterus.

No doctor had ever discovered my problem because the fallopian tubes can't be felt in a pelvic exam unless they're enlarged, and even clubbing doesn't necessarily enlarge them enough to be identified. Since the reproductive organs are nestled in such close proximity, my left tube and ovary were kind of welded together, so webbed with adhesions that the ovary was almost invisible. Craft explained that microsurgery would clear the tubes, but that they would certainly close again within six months—my window of opportunity for getting pregnant. He might have to remove the ovary that looked so severely compromised, but he reassured me that I was perfectly capable of producing a viable egg from the remaining ovary.

It was a dagger blow. For months I'd been on that emotional roller coaster of waiting for my period and feeling utterly demol-ished when I bled, right on schedule. But the clockwork regularity of my cycle left me unprepared to hear this news. I'd never had any menstrual problems, any pain with sex, any indication of the damage in my pelvis, and after months of charting my temperature, I felt a certain intimacy with my reproductive plumbing. I cried bitter, self-indulgent, why-me tears. But I'm also a doctor's daugh-ter, with an inviolate faith in medicine, appeased that technology would provide me with an opportunity not available to an earlier generation.

It was a five-hour surgery. My left ovary and fallopian tube were removed. The other tube was cleared by excising the clubbed end and turning up the edge, like making a skirt hem. My periods resumed right on schedule, but while recuperating, I had an allergic reaction to an antibiotic, which made me break out in hives the size of tangerines. I didn't feel well for quite a while, but I had only six months of possible conception, so Andrew and I embraced the task at hand as if it were a test we had to cram for: lots of winey dinners, lots of peach-colored lingerie, the occasional lunchtime tryst, and three weeks in bucolic Greece. Sex is a glorious thing, when I do it on *my* terms, and this was *not* on my terms. The tacit mandate of procreation made me tense, and the ignominy of lying with my feet in the air afterward made me furious—I kept thinking: People get pregnant doing it in *doorways*. But despite the onus of lust on command, we were randy, uninhibited, energetic, and determined.

Nothing.


I REMEMBERED HEARING about in vitro fertilization just a year before my own problems began. In 1978 the birth of Louise Brown, the first test-tube baby, was front-page news around the world, but particularly in London, since the Brown family and the maverick doctor Patrick Steptoe were British. IVF was truly the stuff of science fiction, something akin to cloning today: augmenting a woman's chance to produce a viable egg with fertility drugs, then harvesting that egg and uniting it with sperm in a petri dish. I certainly shared the public thrill that such a thing was possible, never dreaming it would impinge on my own life. Now, still grieving about my inability to get pregnant in the customary way, I couldn't believe my doctor was saying this unprecedented procedure might work for me.

It was referred to as a "test-tube try," and here's how it would happen: I'd get my period and call the hospital. Then I'd go get my pills, which I'd take on the fifth through ninth days of my cycle. I never fully understood the logic of this routine at the time, but of course that's when the follicle containing the egg is maturing. On the eleventh day, I'd go to the hospital for a sonogram, packing up my dolls and dishes (a Britishism for one's various belongings)

106

in case I needed to spend the night. Later, there were injections instead of pills, with more frequent sonograms and blood drawn to check hormone levels. I remember asking what the pills and shots were, but the names Pergonal and Clomid meant nothing to me at the time. And I would have cheerfully rubbed butter all over my body if told that would help me get pregnant.

An abdominal scan requires a full bladder, and it was always a neat trick to drink the required quart of water and hold it in. Lying on my back in a cotton gown, my stomach smeared with some kind of axle grease, and watching the ultrasound screen, I could see an egg, sometimes two or three, each a snowy little blob against a black background. When they were ready to burst out of their follicles, I'd be taken into the operating room just long enough for the doctor to make two small incisions: one right below my belly button for the laparoscope, the fiberoptic tube that would locate the eggs, and another right above my pelvic bone for a syringe that would aspirate them. Today this procedure is usually unnecessary— the eggs can be identified and retrieved with ultrasound and a fine-needle aspiration through the vagina—but in those days it meant general anesthesia, so I always ate lightly the day before. When I woke up, I'd ask straightaway, "Did you get anything?" Sometimes they'd say, "Yes, Liz, we got three," and they'd go to work in the lab, incubating the eggs in a pink culture medium. Sometimes they'd say, "Sorry, Liz, we'll try again next time," and I'd go home, utterly dejected but striving to remain hopeful. I pinned a sonogram picture of my ovaries on my office bulletin board to help illustrate my regular colloquy on the subject; any discussion of female anatomy drew a large audience in the fashion department.

Because the timing was so critical, the hospital had adjacent rooms for the sonography, the laparoscopy, and the laboratory. Often there were several women waiting in the gynecology ward, our legs in the air (a familiar position for the infertile), our situation dictated by a common plight. Our husbands, meanwhile, were lined up waiting their turn in a little bathroom to produce the necessary sperm. In winter this part of the agenda could not be accomplished at home, because Mother Nature likes nice, warm sperm, and it would be too cold by the time we got to the hospital. Later, as more was learned about the process, some of the failures were attributed to the fact that the sperm was kept at room temperature, not womb temperature. The whole arrangement was so primitive and haphazard—the poor guys didn't even have any *Playboys*. I remember the nurse telling one woman, "We're ready—where is your husband?"

"He can't come," the woman said.

"Why can't he get here?" the nurse asked.

"No," said the woman pointedly, "he can't *come*."

It was all pretty comical, in hindsight. When they did get the sperm, they just sort of put it in the dish, and sometimes the dishes fell to the floor, and sometimes they'd lose the eggs—it was real cottage-industry stuff, and accidents happened. These were the earliest days of fertility treatment and it was uncharted territory. There were no clear guidelines about the optimal time to introduce the sperm to the egg or how long their laboratory courtship should last before returning the fertilized egg to the womb. These days IVF is more sophisticated: The eggs are kept at the same temperature and pH as a woman's body, and the transfer is made forty-eight hours after fertilization, when the egg has divided twice into a four-celled embryo. The amenities have progressed too: Today there are "private facilities" in Professor Craft's London clinic "for the production of semen samples," and there is due concern for the anxiety and embarrassment of the men. But back in the Dark Ages, there was likely to be a sheepish, scarlet-faced husband handing over a jelly jar to an impatient technician, a transaction which had all the decorum of a pizza delivery, and we'd joke about the eggs getting cold. It was black humor, to be sure, but I was living on a knife edge the whole time. Every month I'd wait for the phone to ring, hoping to hear that one of my eggs and one of Andrew's sperm had decided to do a little fertility dance.

Out of nine tries, I got that call only once. It was an indescribable thrill to go back to the hospital and look through a microscope at a tiny embryo: a few shadowy globules clinging together for dear life (literally). I was given a Valium to relax a bit and placed on a bed with my legs elevated (again). The embryo was put in a syringe and inserted through the cervix into my uterus. For twenty-four hours I had to lie flat on my back with my knees up—they were afraid it might slip out, since they didn't know what important step might be skipped in bypassing the fallopian tube, what secretions might help the embryo adhere to the wall of the uterus. I had no idea what was in that pink solution used to marinate the developing egg—it could have been Russian dressing, for all I knew. I later learned that the "glue" was called T-6 and had been used for IVF procedures in mice. It's basically hormones, creating an artificial milieu for the embryo to implant. Otherwise, it would just be menstruated away. Which is what eventually happened. I had a "chemical" pregnancy—the very early stages, enough to confirm with a blood test, but ending in a miscarriage so unremarkable, it just seemed like a heavy period.

Still in my early thirties, I was one of the youngest women involved in the IVF program. As difficult as the experience was for Andrew and me, the older couples had quiet desperation etched on their faces, because the age limit for adoptive parents in Britain was thirty-five for a woman, forty for a man, and this hospital ward was the last-chance saloon for some of them. Even without considering health risks, IVF was a huge emotional gamble because of the high failure rate—only one woman became pregnant during the time I was being treated, but it felt like a communal triumph, because it meant *the procedure worked*. A more onerous problem for me was my rage and jealousy toward anyone having babies the old-fashioned way. I couldn't visit friends who had children or talk about them, and I turned away from strollers and playgrounds. I was godmother to three children and virtually ignored them, sending birthday presents from a safe distance.

One friend, a physician herself, was going through fertility treatment at another hospital and urged me to switch to her doctor, but I had complete faith in Professor Craft. That's what you do: You literally place all your eggs in one basket, believing that this is the guru who will give you your children. The couples under Craft's care even helped launch a fund-raising charity called

INFANT to raise money for his work, with a ball at the Royal Kensington Garden Hotel, where we collected several thousand pounds. Today the lucrative fertility business makes such fund-raising sound archaic and quaint. Craft himself now operates out of an elegant Harley Street townhouse with a fireplace in his office, around the corner from the childhood home of Elizabeth Barrett Browning, another doctor's daughter. But my friend grew impatient with her progress and started upping her own dosage of the drugs, a form of self-abuse available to professionals with prescription pads. She did succeed in having three children, including the twins that often result from fertility treatment, but she went through some major physical changes: Her hair turned frizzy and fell out in patches, and her skin became pale and blotchy. I saw no such changes in myself, but it was impossible to ignore what had happened to her and to wonder whether this tweaking of the natural order didn't bode some ill outcome.

There was an ugly but predictable footnote to fertility treatment in those early days: anger and antagonism toward the doctor who had engineered the first test-tube baby but declined to share his data. (The gist of his research was eventually published posthumously.) "Patrick Steptoe and I never seemed to find great harmony together," Professor Craft said recently. "There was a meeting at the Royal College of Obstetricians and Gynaecologists when the announcement was made about their success, and I remember asking questions, with Steptoe trying to put me down as if I were being silly. I asked: Was there a way to put the embryo back at an earlier stage than four cells, because in monkeys you can transfer embryos that have not even divided and they'll still take. I got a very short reply, as if I were a threat to him. I wasn't trying to threaten him, and I didn't see him as a threat to me either. It seemed sad that he wasn't going to impart all his information. I often wondered if he was hoping for a Nobel Prize, which never happened, or to receive a knighthood, which never came either." Steptoe's reasoning was buried with him in 1988. "The birth of Louise Brown was a major pivotal achievement in fertility, in science, in the world," says Craft. "The *New England Journal of*

*Medicine, Lancet,* the *British Medical Journal*—anybody would have been thrilled to publish it."

The business of assisted reproduction that began with that birth was privately funded, without government support, and the same was true when the United States entered the fray: Although an advisory board for the U.S. Department of Health, Education and Welfare concluded that research in the area was "ethically acceptable," it denied early federal funding, and most of the advances in the field came from Britain, France, and Australia. Now there is virtually a full realm of choices for the infertile. The original IVF procedure allows the implanting of an embryo, a fertilized egg that has begun cell division, but there are more options with clever acronyms, strategies that differ with respect to how far the egg has developed and what part of the woman's reproductive system is malfunctioning: A gamete is an egg that's still a single cell; a zygote is a fertilized egg before cell division begins. With gamete intrafallopian transfer, or GIFT, the eggs that have been obtained through the use of fertility drugs are retrieved, mixed with sperm in a dish, and then transferred into one or both fallopian tubes, in the hope that fertilization will take place in its natural setting. Another procedure, called zygote intrafallopian transfer, or ZIFT, combines IVF and GIFT: The eggs are retrieved, fertilized in a dish, and allowed to begin to develop before they're transferred to the fallopian tubes. Even further down the line is the use of donor eggs from young, healthy women, or surrogate motherhood, which involves borrowing not just an egg but a womb for nine months.

It turned out that the technology of assisted reproduction far outpaced regulations arising from the legal and ethical concerns about this bold experiment. There are so many unanticipated scenarios. What happens if fertility drugs produce six eggs, or twelve, or twenty? Suppose some eggs are frozen and later, after one successful pregnancy, deemed expendable: Should they be destroyed or made available to another woman who needs eggs? How about a woman who has frozen her dead husband's sperm for later use but is opposed by his grown children? And what age limitations, if any, should be set? Is sixty-three too old, as in the case of the California woman who gave birth to her first child in 1997, courtesy of a donated egg? All worthy questions, all unsatisfactorily answered so far. But the unanticipated question that most affected my life was: What might this pushing of the reproductive envelope be doing to my ovaries?

# 8

BEING TOLD I had cancer was not as hard as being told I was infertile. That may sound shocking, but the psychology of infertility is pernicious and crushing. When Professor Craft said I'd never have children, I might have jumped out of the hospital windows if they hadn't been hermetically sealed. It was such a devastating shock. I'm not a spoiled brat, and I was well aware of many blessings: job, husband, extended family, opportunities. But infertility was a terrible wound, a blistering non-achievement. Cancer doesn't feel like a failure—it feels like anomie, catastrophe, requiring a complete review of your existence. You may experience self-pity, but then you get on with it because you must. What you don't understand at the time is that it's not necessarily the end of your life, but the beginning of another chapter.

But infertility is the end of a dream. It's about failing at something fundamental, primal, and essentially female. I didn't have the classic baby lust, I'm not particularly drawn to other people's children, and never in a million years would I have pursued the idea of being a single mother. I also believe that infertile couples who decide *not*

113

to adopt, who move along to happy and productive lives without being parents, are making a wise and mature decision. I never thought of childless couples as sad or self-involved. They seem to have even fuller lives: They're the ones who see all the art exhibits I don't have time for, who catch the plays I miss because I can't get a sitter, who haven't abandoned their friends for child-centric activities. It was only important that I have *Andrew's* child. I thought it would be a wonderful child, that we'd make a great amalgam. My fixation had nothing to do with satisfying my parents or his, or any societal notion of what constitutes a family. But I felt that I was depriving Andrew of a unique opportunity, even though he was completely supportive. He really didn't understand why I had gone all "Mumsy" and kept trying to reassure me that he didn't need children to be fulfilled. That was the message that always came through from Andrew. I don't know how well I would have behaved if he'd been the one with the fertility problem, not me.

I did a lot of second-guessing about my infertility, analyzing all the what-ifs and should-haves of my life. Suppose I had cut back at the office, or stopped working altogether and devoted myself full-time to the pursuit of pregnancy? The truth is, I think such a folly would have ended in madness and divorce. I am not a nice person when I'm not busy—in fact, I'm a nightmare. In my darkest moments, it was always good to return to the office. Infertility sucks the pleasure out of your world, eclipsing all the joyful context of wanting a child in the first place. Having a job to do, a place where I had responsibilities and accomplishments while I was so thwarted in another arena, was my salvation.

Andrew did not want to adopt, citing the obvious reservations that it was too hard and took too long. He proposed that we'd have a great time spoiling *other* people's kids and indulging ourselves. I felt there was more subtext to his objections, which he denied: The Greeks in London have a fierce pride of family and culture that would bias him against anything but a biological child. But I also knew that he has a big, soft, generous heart, that his nurturing instincts could be nudged. And so, in early 1980, I embarked on a solitary quest, keeping Andrew in the dark until I phoned him one day in Eastbourne to tell him what I'd been doing.

Private adoption was way beyond our meager budget: It would have required going outside the country, since third-party adoption has been illegal in Britain since 1975. A small number of adoptions are handled through agencies affiliated with the Catholic church. (There was a moment when I considered that my maiden name of Kelly might come in handy. I was also completely prepared to be "Mrs. Rabinowitz.") But few avenues are available to the average Anglican. Most adoptions were and are under the jurisdiction of the Department of Social Services in each borough of the city concerned. I wrote to the director of every borough of every city I'd ever lived in—Manchester, Bath, Leeds—eight in all. Although I knew of no other couples who'd adopted children, I was aware of the difficulties involved from articles I'd read, and I was leaving no stone unturned. Seven of the boroughs wrote back saying that I didn't qualify because I wasn't a resident. The London borough where we did live at the time informed me that there was a long waiting list for white babies, that the only children available were "mixed race." Suddenly I had an inspiration: I could make the case that we had a mixed *marriage.*

Andrew thought I was out of my mind, but I knew that half the battle with adoption was getting the social workers interested in our situation, working on our behalf. Once they'd actually come to our home and petted our cat and sipped from our teacups, they were much more likely to take a personal, proprietary interest in helping us to find a child. My tactic was to convince them that our marriage crossed racial boundaries, a notion that would otherwise have been abhorrent to me, veering too close to my father's early attitude toward Andrew, when he acted as if I were marrying a Martian. But the Greeks born in Britain did constitute a separate and unique culture, mostly living in an enclave near our apartment in Child's Hill, as self-contained a community as the Asians or Middle Easterners in London. And so I played the race card with the Social Services people, without actually specifying what "races" we were talking about.

A social worker was on the phone within twenty-four hours. I had to do a major song and dance to convince Mrs. Rachel Goodman that we constituted a "mixed" couple, and even though she never conceded that point, she insisted that Greek people never give up children for adoption. She also let us know that a black infant would almost certainly go to a black couple and an Indian infant to an Indian couple. Just because Andrew had a swarthy complexion and an exotic lineage didn't mean we were likely to get a dark-skinned baby any time soon.

Friends who've adopted children in the United States sometimes talk about "pulling rank" and getting themselves moved to the top of a waiting list, but the British system is different. It really is a meritocracy. The Social Services are concerned with finding a family for a child, not the other way around. Mrs. Goodman turned out to be a formidable, matronly lady with a deep, warm voice and darkly graying hair, who gave the distinct impression that she would brook no nonsense. There was no mistaking that her priority was the children entrusted to her care. From the first interview, she let us know in many subtle and tacit ways that the only criterion she was interested in was that we were worthy, deserving, and capable parents, according to standards we might never have anticipated. Years later, she told us about visiting a potential adoptive couple whose home was so pristine that she worried about their adjusting to the disorder of a child. One day she asked to use the bathroom in their home, and when she got to the second floor of the house, she was delighted to find it a mess.

I didn't have any worries about our home being too perfect. We had a rather bare-bones apartment before minimalism was chic—sleeping in my parents' hand-me-down bed and shopping for furniture in junk shops, with a few modern pieces of Andrew's design. I had made all the curtains, from inexpensive fabrics—buying readymade rings and poles to hang them was a real extravagance. We had no washer or dryer, and all our clothes fitted into one old wardrobe. It wasn't an apartment that would have given Mrs. Goodman any cause for concern. But we realized that she would be judging us as a couple, ascertaining whether we had a strong marriage despite all the traveling back and forth and despite

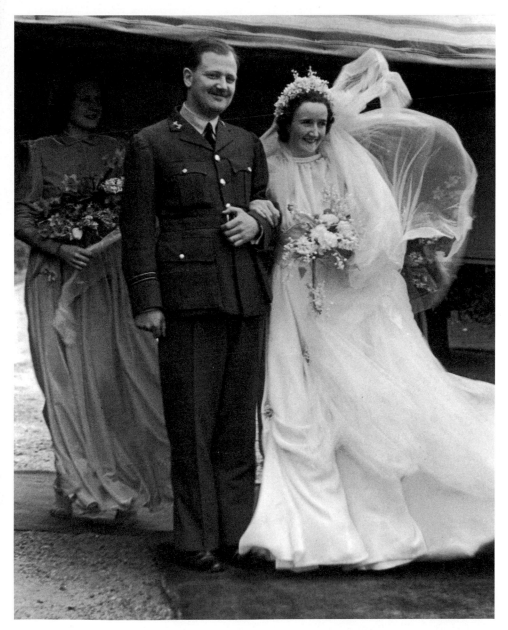

The day that my father, Thomas Stuart-Black Kelly, married my mother, Janet Caldwell—February 20, 1940. He's dressed in his Royal Air Force uniform, as he had already been called up into service; Mummy is wearing an ivory velvet wedding dress `caught up with tiny bunches of ivory orange blossoms (in Alderley Edge in Cheshire).

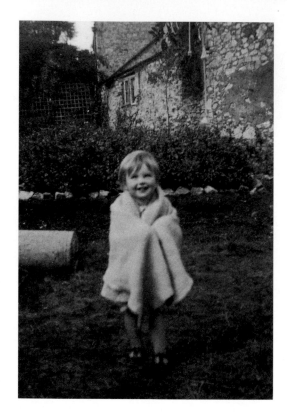

"Blanket-round-downstairs!" My never-ending desire to be the life of the party, in the garden at Shirehampton, summer 1950.

"Penn-y-Bryn"—The house on the hill in Hereford with its fabulous fairy-tale garden, where we moved when I was three.

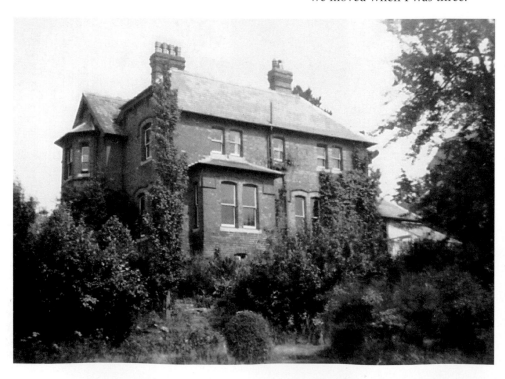

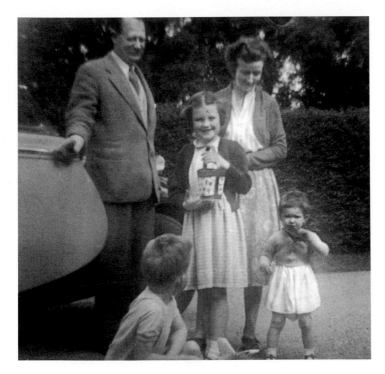

Family complete:
Mummy; Daddy;
my brother, Grant;
me; and my sister,
Lois.

The Jaguar that
Daddy converted
into a station
wagon, in which
we toured America
in 1957.

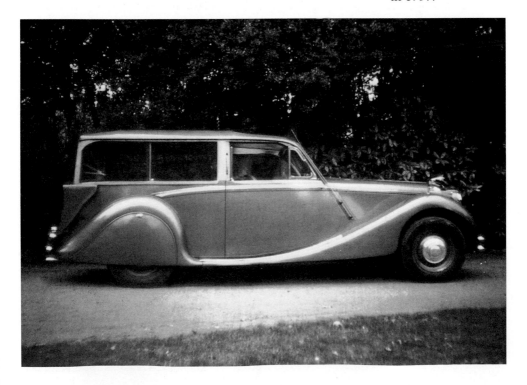

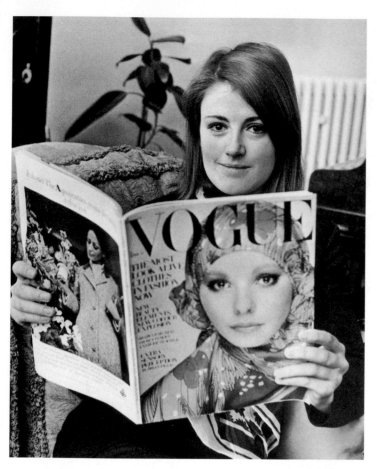

The beginning of my career: after I won the *Vogue* talent contest, this picture appeared in the *Bath and Wiltshire Evening Chronicle*. Note my Celia Birtwell scarf peeking out from beneath the *Vogue* cover.

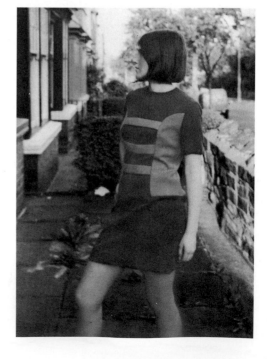

Modeling my first designs at Leicester Polytechnic in 1965.

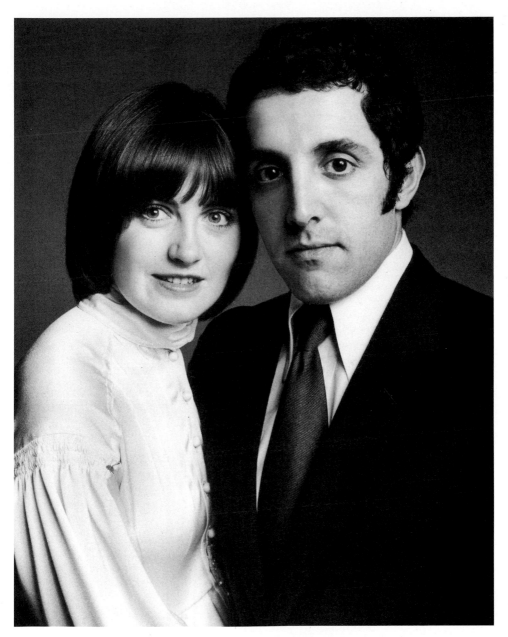

My official wedding portrait with my husband, Andrew, by Barry Lategan in 1971. My dress is by Jean Muir; the bridegroom wore brown.

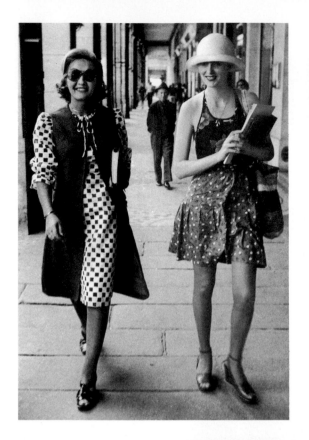

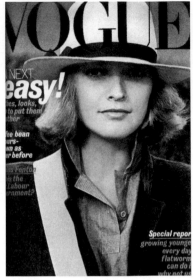

The very first British *Vogue* cover
I ever styled. Kirsti Moseng, now
Toscani, photographed by her
husband-to-be, Oliviero Toscani.
August 1977.

My mentors:
Beatrix Miller, then editor-
in-chief of British *Vogue*,
and Grace Coddington,
then fashion editor, walking in Paris in the early
1970s. *(Photo courtesy of
Grace Coddington.)*

With the wonderful Sheila
Wetton, fashion editor of
British *Vogue*, taken by
Arthur Elgort during a
sitting at Chiswick House,
around 1973.
*(Photo by Arthur Elgort.)*

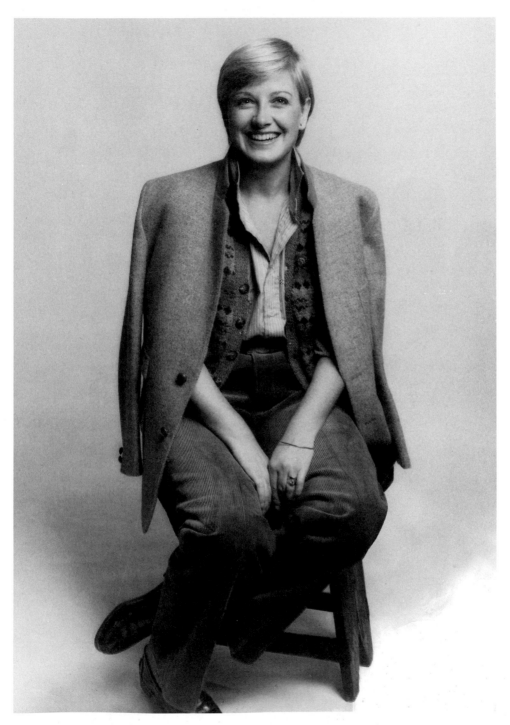

My dear friend the late Terence Donovan took this picture of me, and it was published in British *Vogue* in a section called "In Their Own Fashion" along with photos of Sheila Wetton and Grace Coddington in November 1977. All clothes by Margaret Howell.

With Bruce Weber,
photographed by
Tim Geaney, on our
first trip together, to
Greece, in 1979.

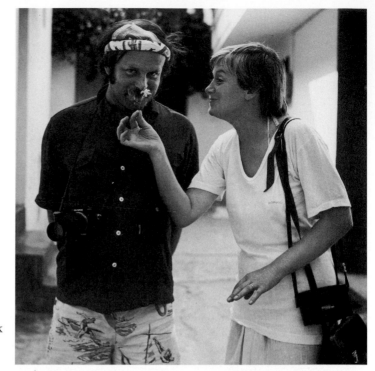

On location on
Hampstead Heath in
August 1980 with
Terry May (second
from left) and Patrick
Demarchelier (far
right).

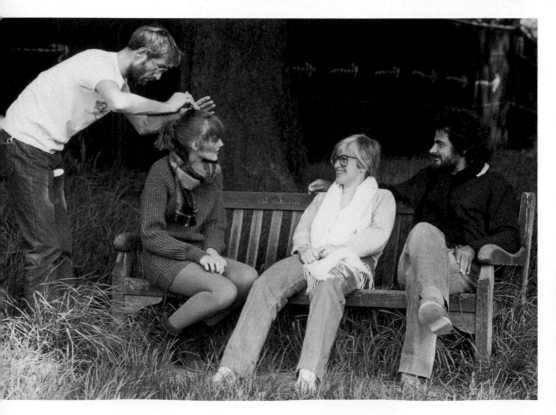

Proud parent: holding
Robert on his first visit
home in July 1981.

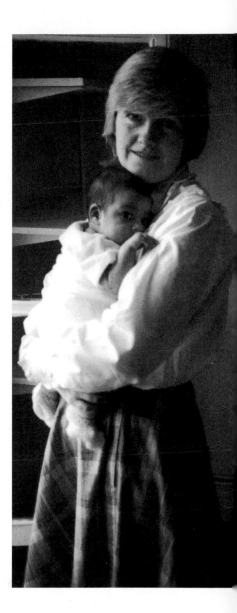

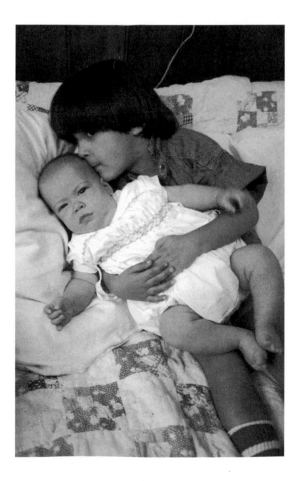

Robbie hugs his new
brother, Christopher,
March 1985.

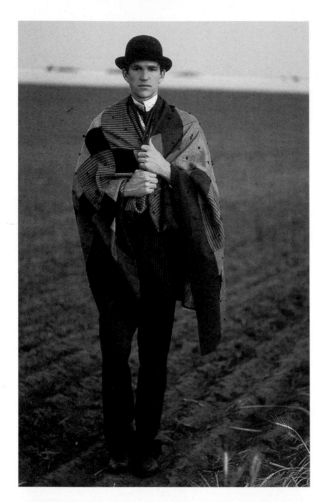

Nebraska 1981—
Matthew Modine, the
actor, becomes a pioneer
on Bruce Weber's
Willa Cather–inspired
shoot. *(Photo by Bruce
Weber.)*

Matt Dillon in the location
van with Bruce Weber.

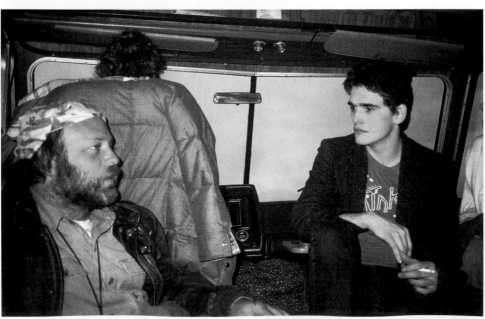

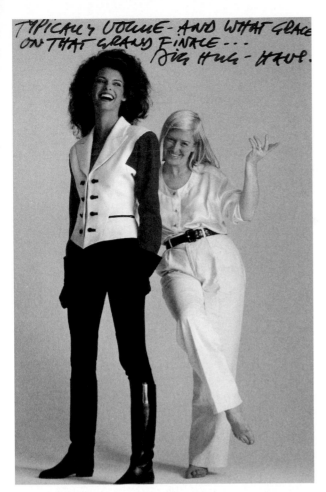

*TYPICALLY VOGUE - AND WHAT GRACE ON THAT GRAND FINALE... BIG HUG - HANS.*

My last sitting with photographer Hans Feurer before I became editor-in-chief of British *Vogue* in 1987. Linda Evangelista (before her famous haircut) and me on the set.

Robbie and me in an advertisement for GapKids on a London double-decker bus in 1987, while I was editor-in-chief of British *Vogue*.

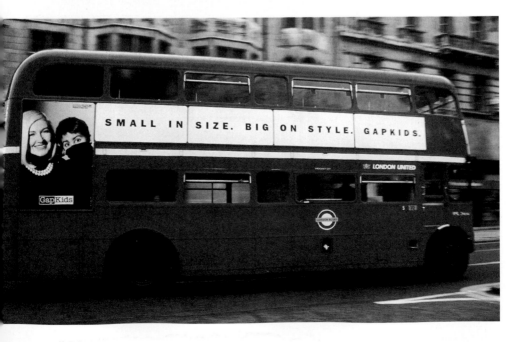

SMALL IN SIZE. BIG ON STYLE. GAPKIDS.

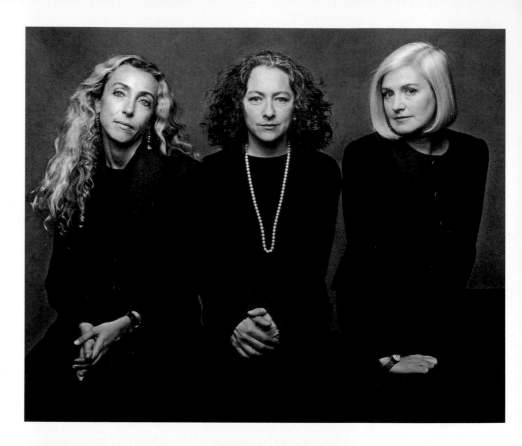

The European editors
of *Vogue:* from left,
Franca Sozzani of
Italian *Vogue*, Irene
Silvani of French *Vogue*,
and me. *(Photo by
Patrick Demarchelier.)*

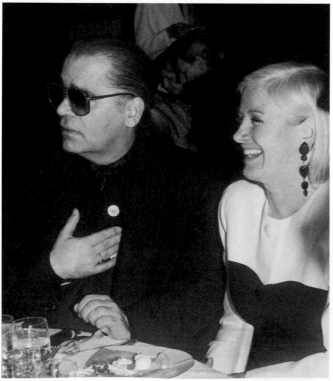

Karl Lagerfeld and me
having a fun-filled chat
at an AIDS fund-raising
dinner in Paris in 1988.
*(Photo by Dave Benett.)*

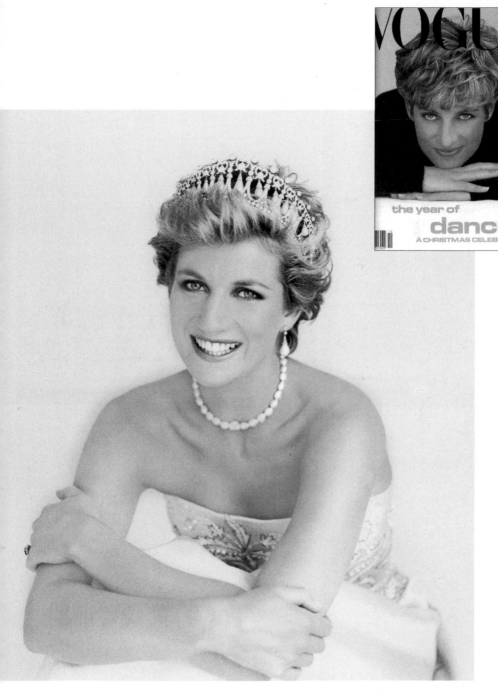

The eternally famous tiara pictures of Her Royal Highness the Princess of Wales, photographed for the December 1990 issue of British *Vogue*.
*(Photo by Patrick Demarchelier.)*

*(inset)* The cover for which the princess and I had always hoped—December 1991.
*(Photo by Patrick Demarchelier.)*

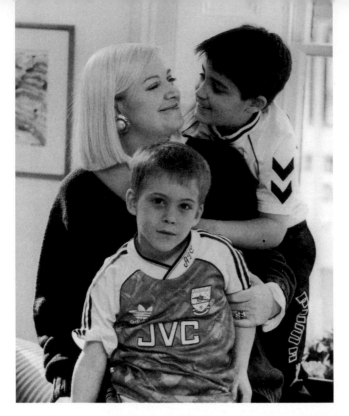

The boys in their football uniforms and me in the St. John's Wood house in London, taken by Michel Arnaud.

My last evening in the UK was a fund-raiser for AIDS. Here, my two children present flowers to Her Royal Highness the Princess of Wales at the *Prince of Tides* premiere. March 1992. *(Photo by Richard Young.)*

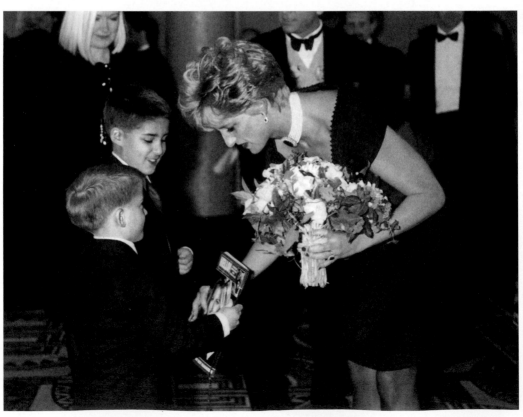

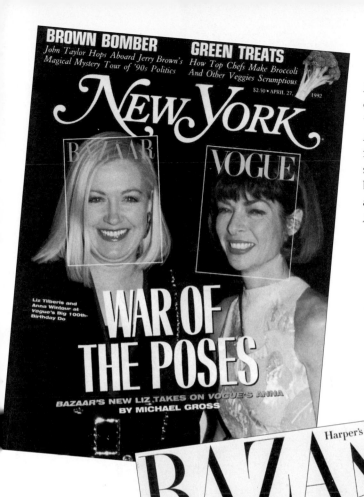

New York magazine cover, April 27, 1992— "War of the Poses." Anna Wintour and I featured in the cover story on the competition between *Harper's Bazaar* and *Vogue*. *(Photo by Mary Hilliard.)*

The first issue of the new era: September 1992. Linda Evangelista as photographed by Patrick Demarchelier.

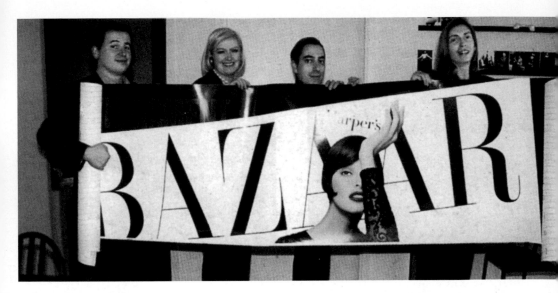

The creative team with the bus posters for our first cover. From left: creative director Fabien Baron, me, and fashion directors Paul Cavaco and Tonne Goodman. *(Photo courtesy of Hearst Magazine.)*

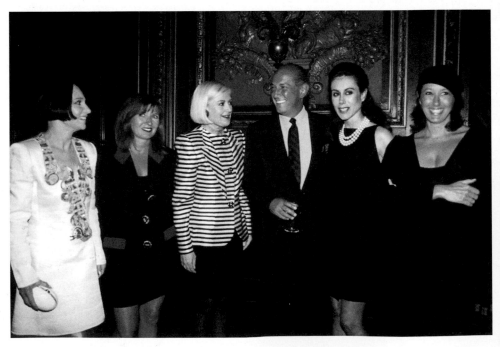

The launch party for the September issue at the Metropolitan Club in New York. With me, from left to right, are designers Mary McFadden, Nicole Miller, Oscar de la Renta, Carolyne Roehm, and Donna Karan. *(Photo courtesy of Hearst Magazine.)*

all that we had been through in our infertility trauma, that Andrew didn't beat me and I didn't cheat on him, that we could support a child financially, that we were caring people capable of getting our hands dirty, that we had parenting skills or could learn them.

It's hard to demonstrate a talent for marriage or parenthood to a total stranger. There's a certain self-consciousness about where to sit, how and when to touch each other, what to wear or say. There is the dichotomy of being on your best behavior while seeming effortlessly at ease. Andrew and I didn't attempt to "prepare," except for our position on religious training, which we'd decided to do without. We'd discuss God endlessly, and if our child wanted to be Catholic or Muslim or Zoroastrian, no problem— we'd support any religious choice. But we wouldn't agree to specific demands about religion from the birth parents. Beyond that, we knew we had to stand on our own merits. Ultimately we realized that the social worker had probably seen it all and couldn't be suckered. Most important, we had nothing to hide. We loved each other and wanted to share that love with a child. Although Andrew had started out diffident and detached, there's a moment in a caring marriage when one spouse realizes what is important to ensure the other's happiness and goes along, sometimes embracing the idea so fully that it eclipses the earlier doubt, which is what happened with us.

I did tell one gigantic lie: I said I had fulfilled all my career goals and wanted to stay home with my baby. In later years, Mrs. Goodman told me those words were graven on her heart as she watched my behemoth ambition come to fruition, but I was desperate enough to say anything.

There were many visits, all part of the ongoing vetting process to ensure that we were consistent in what we said and did, and each one preceded by an episode of self-flagellation or reproach— were we showing ourselves to be bright enough, determined enough, easygoing, thoughtful, judicious, reasonable, happy? Mrs. Goodman was pleased with our support system of grandparents at the ready, and she was interested in our rejecting the tradition of boarding school at an early age. (Yes, I'd loved it myself, but I wasn't going to all that effort just to relinquish my child to a headmaster for most of the year.) She tried to reveal all the tripwires of adoption, warn us of all the difficulties. Over and over again, she impressed upon us the possibility that an adopted child might come from a background different from any we knew, that his parents were not likely to be rocket scientists and that he might never be academically gifted or even bright. Andrew and I thought this was hogwash: A lot of the talented, artistic people we knew came from humble beginnings, and we were quite sure that *our* child would be brilliant—the classic nature-versus-nurture debate.

She was also looking, as we found out after the fact, for the earmarks of maturity. Deciding to become parents is one thing, but parenting another person's child takes a different kind of pluck and resolve and something she called "stickability." Social workers understand that even the most straightforward adoption of the healthiest baby still involves a child who has already had a setback, and been disadvantaged from the start: The birth mother was probably not too cheerful during her pregnancy, and the baby could have suffered instant rejection. Mrs. Goodman had seen babies turn to the wall in their cribs, traumatized and unresponsive. She needed to warn us that the most adorable baby can become a snarling, truculent teenager who uses adoption as a cudgel ("Don't tell me what to do—you're not even my real father!"). Despite these conversations, I finally relaxed about her visits and chats, about how the pillows were arranged on the couch or what kind of tea I served, but the initial trepidation about being "suitable" was replaced by a lingering anxiety over whether we would get a baby at all.

About six months after our first meeting, in May 1981, I was working at my desk, getting ready to accompany Bruce Weber to Nebraska for the Willa Cather shoot, when Mrs. Goodman called. "Are you sitting down?" she said. "Robbie is here." Robbie's mother was a young English woman who worked in a print shop, and his father was an Iranian who had deserted her when she became pregnant. This young woman had been brought up by her father after her mother died, and she didn't want her own child to grow up with only one parent. Robbie was placed with a foster family just outside London, but his mother was still visiting him. She was certain that she wouldn't keep him, but she wanted him to know, even on an unconscious level, as some tactile memory, that his mother had cared about him and cuddled him as an infant. The Social Services department encouraged that kind of attention. They wanted to increase the possibility that the natural mother would decide to keep her own baby. And even if she didn't change her mind and allowed the adoption to proceed, they were keen for the baby to have some early motherlove and attention.

The first time we were allowed to see Robbie, he was a month old. We drove behind the social worker to a council estate in Edgware—low-cost public housing in small semi-detached frame homes built after World War II. Most of the fenced-in yards were neat and clean, but as we drove farther and farther into the estate, we came upon a yard that looked like a junk shop, piled high with old porcelain bathtubs, iron bits and pieces. I felt my stomach sink when Mrs. Goodman's car stopped in front of this house, but my qualms disappeared when I met the foster family, who were warm and loving people, the father a plumber and the mother bringing up several children of their own. Robbie was on a big brown sofa. He was tiny and dark, with black hair and shining brown eyes, wearing an awful green cardigan with red and yellow flowers, and he howled the whole time we were there. But my heart skipped a beat the moment I saw him. I touched each of his fingers and toes, counting them several times, reveling in the silk of his skin, and when he grasped a strand of my hair as I bent over him, I began to weep—huge, cleansing, grateful, triumphant sobs. It was like winning all the money in the world. I think my husband was even more overwhelmed, because it was obvious from the moment we saw Robbie that this was how any child fathered by Andrew actually might look. Robbie was our son, but we still had to jump through hoops to prove it.

Every day for several weeks I'd leave work early and drive to see him. His foster mother and I would take him for walks, and she'd talk to me about babies—I knew nothing about preparing formula or changing diapers or giving him a bath. Pregnant mothers have nine months to begin bonding with a child, but Robbie and I had a different sort of courtship. Finally his foster mother started urging me to take him home for visits—she said he was beginning to realize that there were two maternal faces looking at him, and she was worried that he'd have a hard time leaving her. I was terrified, certain that he would drop and break in my care. I brought him home on a Saturday afternoon, and Grace Coddington came over to double the population of novices who knew nothing about babies. Every time he cried, we changed his diaper, going through an easy dozen in one day (the cloth kind that have to be soaked and washed). But that first visit broke the ice, not the baby. Andrew tried to get him to watch a soccer game on TV, and I tried to hold him up to the telephone for my mother to say hello, and I thought I'd die when I had to relinquish him back to foster care at the end of the day. I felt the grief of his birth mother, cutting out part of her heart to give him a better life. I was overwhelmed with love and fear about being entrusted with his welfare. The next weekend, he slept overnight with us, in the crib from my own infancy (I'd stolen it from my mother and stored it all those years). By July he was with us full-time. I have pictures of Robbie on Andrew's knee, with the wedding of Lady Diana Spencer and Prince Charles on TV in the background.

Up until November, when we went before the judge in Willesden County Court and finalized the adoption, Robbie's birth mother could have come forward to claim him, but I never even contemplated that possibility. Apparently she lived not far from us, and the social workers feared she would have second thoughts if she saw a rather pale woman walking around with an olive-skinned little boy. But I wasn't concerned. If she had come up to me on the street and said, "That must be my baby," I would have said, "Well, yes, he probably is." I was very un-paranoid about the fact that somebody else had given birth to him. By that time, Robbie was so much our son. We fell in love with him so quickly and felt secure that he was going to be ours forever. That is my particular forte: When I hit on a focused, optimistic point of view, nothing can deter me.

It was a bitter wintry day when it became legal, the weather too inclement and the distance too great for our parents to travel. Robbie was dressed in Oshkosh jeans, and the judge commented on what a handsome fellow he was. I was petrified that he would say, "Of course, Mrs. Tilberis, you're going to stop work, immediately and forever," that he would declare me an unfit mother because I was returning to a full-time job in six months. But the courtroom formality is a gentle procedure, with a lot of dignity and due consideration given to the fact that most people in this situation have been little exposed to legal machinations and might find the experience intimidating. When such a momentous event is happening, you might expect fireworks, epiphanies, an acknowledgment that something *big* has transpired. But it was all pretty matter-of-fact. No champagne celebration: We just gave each other a hug, and then it was time to take Robbie home for lunch in his high chair. We never met his birth mother: That was Andrew's choice. With his art background, my husband is a visual person, and he didn't want to have an image of her in his head every time he looked at our son. I didn't question his reasoning or argue the point—it wasn't that important to me. The only important thing was having Robbie.

My family heaved a collective sigh of relief when they saw me settled as a mother. They knew I was determined to have a baby by hook or by crook, and the "crook" part had seemed a distinct possibility. My brother, who was completing his medical training, had been married the same weekend we first learned about Robbie, and Andrew and I sat through the wedding festivities with Cheshire cat grins on our faces, not wanting to distract attention from the bride and groom on their big day. They were among the first visitors to our new family, after their honeymoon. But my sister had to leap tall buildings to come see her first nephew: Lois had been recruited straight from high school into MI6, Her Majesty's Secret Service. Until her retirement several years ago, she led a rather cryptic and covert life. We never knew much or asked much about her whereabouts and responsibilities—part of a tacit bargain made in the family of someone doing classified government work. If my parents were questioned about her, they answered with innocuous vagueness, making their daughter sound like a bureaucrat or pencil-pusher. Since she was not married and had no children of her own, Lois cheerfully accepted the role of Auntie, swooping down for impromptu visits. She'd call (on her shoe phone, for all I knew) from a low-flying helicopter over the North Sea and say, "I'm ten minutes away." Very dramatic, but we got used to it.

I felt secure enough at *Vogue* that a six-month sabbatical wouldn't jeopardize my chances for advancement, and Grace was a great booster. I'd always been so envious of colleagues who brought their children to work, seeing Bea making a fuss. (She was quite good with little ones, getting down on her hands and knees, if necessary, to play.) But despite my excitement, I didn't take Robbie in to show off at *Vogue* right away—the office seemed too dirty, and I had the typical new mother's phobia about exposing the baby to germs. I also wasn't prepared for the exhaustion of going *anywhere* with an infant. Toting trunks of clothes to fashion sittings all those years was nothing compared to climbing four flights of stairs with a pram and bags of baby paraphernalia every time I left the house, mostly on my own, as Andrew was still commuting to the restaurant during the week.

When maternity leave was up, I was ready to go back to work and Andrew was prepared to stay home, having resigned his lectureship at Leeds the previous year, and that's the way it's been ever since. My husband's ego was big enough to encompass the idea of being Mr. Mom—he saw it as role enhancement, rather than role reversal. He had despaired of ever supporting the family with his artwork, unwilling to make the sort of compromises that might have facilitated commercial success, and teaching wasn't very lucrative either. Andrew had gone back and earned a bachelor of arts education degree at London University, but he didn't enjoy the bureaucratic and political sides of academia—carrying a briefcase, jockeying for tenure. He had also been frustrated in his attempts to ensure the continuation of a certain kind of education for British art students. Working with the National Standing Conference for Foundation Education in Art and Design, he had gathered statistics demonstrating that when art students were allowed to take the kind of "pre-dip" course that I'd taken—experiencing various subjects before selecting a degree program—they ultimately found more professional success in their chosen field. But Margaret Thatcher, then minister of education, wanted to do away with pre-dip, which she considered an unnecessary luxury.

Finding himself happier at home than he'd ever expected to be and grateful to have time with our son, Andrew set his mind on the course of full-time fatherhood. He sold his restaurant in 1981 and decided mine was the career that could at this time take precedence. It's an unconventional arrangement that has always worked for us, and I do think that an early bonding experience with a strong father figure may have a felicitous effect on a boy's development. But I was an endlessly guilty working mother. The guilt starts the moment you hold the child. When you're at work, you're thinking about the baby, and when you're at home, you're thinking about why you can't think about work because you're thinking about the baby. I'd decided that *my* child wasn't going to eat packaged foods, so I'd spend weekends making purées out of cauliflower and carrots (only to find them defiantly turned to mold in a corner of the refrigerator). Leaving the house in the morning was a heartbreak, wanting to go back for one last cuddle, sure that Robbie would love Andrew more than me. As he got older, I couldn't even have a kiss goodbye, because he'd start to cry when he realized I would be gone for the day, so I had to distract him with toys and sneak out.

Despite my early concerns for his safety, Robbie got through his childhood unscathed—but Andrew didn't. When the baby was about a year old, we went to my parents' house in Bath for a long weekend while they were vacationing in the Lake District. On a very hot Sunday afternoon in July, Andrew decided to burn a huge heap of leaves and garden debris that my father had left piled on the lawn. He went down to the cellar and got a canister labeled

123

kerosene, which would ignite and burn in a controlled manner. In fact, it held gasoline. I watched what happened next as if it were in slow motion: Andrew, wearing only a bathing suit, struck a match and bent over the pile to light it. The air was still that day, and the fumes sort of sat on top of the bonfire for a moment, then shot up like a bomb. A ball of fire descended, licking his face, arms, chest, and legs. He looked like a stuntman in a movie, his body covered with leaping flames. I grabbed the blanket I was sitting on and threw it over him, then raced into the house and called 999 for an ambulance. There were high sandstone pillars at the gate of the house, and the ambulance driver had a hard time maneuvering around them. "Can your husband walk?" he called to me. Andrew appeared at that moment like something out of a bog, an apparition in red and black, his charred skin falling off like torn clothes, covered in the newly mown grass and pine needles that he had rolled in trying to put the flames out. "Never mind," said the driver quickly, "we're coming in."

The nearest hospital, the Royal United, was not equipped to treat him, but by purest serendipity, there was an excellent burn unit not far away at the Frenchay Hospital, constructed of Nissen huts, prefabricated in corrugated steel, during World War II. Although he looked monstrous, the doctors assured me that the burns were superficial and he would be home, unscarred, in two weeks. Every day I'd drive to see him, a mummy wrapped in white from head to toe, waiting in the window and stiffly waving his arm slowly from side to side in greeting. He screamed every day when he had a bath, but two weeks later, as promised, the bandages were removed, and his skin was enviably smooth and unlined, the fire having achieved a do-it-yourself dermabrasion. To this day, he doesn't have any wrinkles. I hate him.


WHEN I WENT back to British *Vogue* after maternity leave, I was scared. The fashion business is all about a feeling for the moment. You can lose it in a week, and I'd been gone six months. But fashion was in a wild mode then, and I was made for the over-the-topness of it. I look back on what Grace and I were doing in the early 1980s, and I'm astonished. Our pages were a high-wire act that narrowly avoided toppling into pure eccentricity. I wonder now how Beatrix Miller ever let us get away with it: faces doused in powder paint, hair set in plaster, yellow lips, red eyes, clothes that were upside down, inside out, full of holes, lashed together with bondage straps. The designers created the clothes, and we accentuated the look, endorsing and enhancing the runway images with ideas taken from the street and the art colleges. (Britain is riddled with art colleges.) The great romance with sleek Americana continued but made room for the wearable Japanese sculpture of Issey Miyake, for the highly sexed second skins of Azzedine Alaia, for the transported club scene of Rifat Ozbek. It was a fashion cataclysm—our taste was revolutionized. It was nothing for John Galliano to present a homage to Pearly Kings and Queens, for Jean Paul Gaultier to do absurd conical bras spiraling toward the ceiling, or for Didier Malige to style hair that looked like a stack of twigs or white dreadlocks.

I was definitely out there, even more so than Grace, who always stayed on the romantic side of things, never going as far as I did with black fingers and spiky chains in hair, and she never espoused the Japanese as ardently, so I didn't have to fight her for a trip to Japan in 1984. We took the bullet train from Tokyo to Kyoto and stayed in a *ryokan* (a traditional Japanese inn) that was Marlon Brando's home when he made *The Teahouse of the August Moon*; we slept on tatami mats and ate in sushi bars, where there was a welcoming line of salt on the floor. In Kanazawa we were shooting from a converted warship on the Sea of Japan; abalone and other delicacies were retrieved for our dinner by sea divers. But "round eyes" aren't accustomed to seafood brought back from such a great depth, we discovered. I broke out in hives, the Japanese version of Montezuma's revenge.

The paradigm of the model for this period was Uma Thurman or Kristen McMenamy, odd-looking beauties in great quantities of fabric, like Turkish pants so voluminous that we dubbed them

125

"seven-day shits"—the amount that could be concealed within the folds. (I keep telling you: The fashion business isn't pretty.) The image wasn't exactly about clothes anyone could wear. In one mad moment, the caption for a model wearing Galliano and a pair of broken spectacles gave the useful tip, "First, smash your glasses." We broke all the rules and worked against the literal, evoking eighteenth-century dandies with extraordinary hair that tumbled and snaked. Heads were bound up with cloth and tulle to look like medieval headdresses from a Vermeer painting. It was about historical references, beautiful images, nothing to do with women at the end of the twentieth century. But fashion photography isn't necessarily about real people. The idea was (and still is, for that matter) to get people into the stores to buy clothes—that is the point of magazines. It's about romance, fantasy, cutting edge, moving on. We're dragging the reader along with us and saying: You can't wear the same camel coat for the rest of your life.

The most extreme work I ever did was with the Scottish photographer Albert Watson. For one sitting, I used a six-foot tall, rawboned, androgynous beauty named Lynn Koestler, matted her hair and eyebrows with silver paint, whitened her lips, and dressed her in a rubber knee-length dress with two-inch nails protruding from her chest, worn under a sheath of barbed wire, from a shop called Fetish or Die in the Kensington Antiques Market. The zenith of that esoteric phase came when Watson shot the August 1984 cover with Talisa Soto's lips smeared with purple, yellow, and silver, and a rock over one eye. Rocks and rubber? The look didn't reflect me or anyone I knew. But the work was about dazzle, about excitement and inspiration, extending the boundaries of style, the adventure of adorning ourselves. It was not about what my colleagues and I wore. You wouldn't believe how conservative the personal style of some fashion editors is. A few prominent authorities do not seem to have changed styles since VE Day, and one of them looks very like an aging Wilma Flintstone. When I left the studio, I was a white-haired mum nearing forty, running alongside a toddler on a tricycle in the park and thinking about adopting another baby.

ONCE YOU'VE ADOPTED a child in Britain, you stand a good chance of getting another, because the Social Services are keen on children growing up in "traditional" homes with siblings. Their studies show that two adopted children in a family do better than one. I continued to have "test-tube tries," hoping to become one of the proverbial cases of women who adopt one child and then "relax" and conceive on their own. Mrs. Goodman was more practical. When she made one of her periodic visits, she'd gently prod us about getting on the waiting list to adopt again. Ultimately even my dogged optimism gave out, and we made a formal application. But it wasn't until July 1985 that Christopher became our son.

When the phone rang this time, it was the social worker for a sixteen-year-old English girl whose premature baby boy had been living for nearly three months in the pediatric ICU of Edgware General Hospital. His lungs were not fully developed, and he had stopped breathing right after he was born, so the doctors still weren't sure what harm might have been done before he was resuscitated. Oxygen deprivation can cause blindness, deafness, even brain damage.

"Quite frankly," I said, "we're not interested." I'm not proud of it, but in my heart I could not imagine undertaking the care of a mentally handicapped child. There are people who do, and I think they are probably saints on earth, but I don't have that kind of soul. If such a child were born to me, I hope I'd have the fortitude to cope and give him the best possible opportunities, but taking on such misfortune willingly seemed unimaginable. And if this child had such special needs, I thought he should go to the sort of magnificent people who can embrace such a challenge.

Social Services were not pleased with me. It was obvious they thought I was acting like a princess who wanted to be presented with a perfect child on a silver platter. And I suppose their censure, however tacit, had its effect. I called the social worker back and said we'd like to have the baby examined to determine the extent of his injuries and requirements. That was fine with the agency as long as we paid the expenses.

127

So Chris was taken by his foster mother to an ophthalmologist at the National Institute, and a neurologist at Middlesex Hospital, and finally a pediatrician at Queen Charlotte's—all top physicians whom my father helped us find. Miraculously, everyone sent a good report. There was nothing physically, neurologically, or mentally wrong that couldn't be fixed with loving care and attention. The pediatrician called me as soon as Chris had left his office to say, "This is probably the most normal child I've ever held in my life." We were on the phone to the social worker in a flash, staking our claim.

We still hadn't seen him. I knew I couldn't have walked away from a child I'd actually held in my arms—no woman could, I suspect—so we didn't visit him until the medical tests were complete.

A virus had infiltrated the ICU where Chris was tended as a newborn before he was well enough to go into foster care, and he hadn't been cuddled all that time. Those first three months of his life had been lonely ones. We could see that as soon as we looked at him. Chris was quite solemn, not the strong and spirited baby Robbie had been, with a pale moon face, completely expressionless, like a block of wood. We petted him and snuggled with him and tried to charm him, but he seemed to have virtually no interest in us. Then Andrew and I went down to the local pub, where I ordered a large sherry and started to cry. I was sure he was sick and we were on the brink of disaster. But Andrew said we were simply looking at a very young baby who hadn't really woken up yet. The foster parents were sweet but much older, and their home was a quiet place, dull and gray, no visual stimulation at all except for a TV. Chris was in a room all by himself. "I think if I were living in that house," said Andrew, "I'd look just like him."

The next day at work, I told Beatrix Miller that I was about to bring home an infant and needed a month off. Shockingly, she got furious with me and made no attempt to conceal her anger from the rest of the staff. My colleagues made me a card that said, "Congratulations on Christopher. *We* still love you." Looking back, I think I must have caught her completely off guard, because she was a gracious woman who would never have tried to sabotage my happiness. But adoption doesn't give new parents or anyone in their orbit much time to prepare: We were bringing Chris home the next day. In tears, I called my mother, who said, "Go to the store and buy what you need"—shopping as therapy. I decided Christopher deserved a brand-new, state-of-the-art baby carriage. A saleswoman told me that the hot color in prams was black. Fine with me—it would match all my clothes.

"But I want it delivered right away," I said.

"When is the baby due?" she asked quizzically, eyeing my figure, which was not obviously pregnant.

"Tomorrow," I chirped, and she looked at me like I was mad.

That afternoon, I started preparing four-year-old Robbie for the fact that he was getting a brother the next day. Kids are so agreeable and defenseless about matters that flummox adults. He wasn't distressed that Mummy didn't have a big stomach for nine months, that he hadn't listened to the baby's heartbeat or painted the nursery blue. And he came with us to the foster home the next day to pick up Chris. Robbie took one look at the serious baby, walked over to the crib, and tickled him. And Christopher burst out laughing—maybe for the first time in his life. The child was literally shivering with love, completely transformed, in a split second, by his brother. It was a gorgeous thing.

A few months later, we went to the same courthouse where Robbie's adoption had been formalized to sign similar reams of paper for Chris. Each of our sons has his birth mother's surname as part of his name, and they know why. We've always been completely relaxed and candid about their backgrounds—when Robbie was a toddler and couldn't quite get a handle on the word "adopted," he used to go around claiming, "I'm a doctor." But sometimes people would ask in a hushed and concerned voice, "Are you going to tell him?" It seems like an obsolete question now, but in the 1980s the subject of adoption was still cloaked with some secrecy, embarrassment, and stigma. Today there is nothing extraordinary about Caucasians adopting a child from China or Korea or anywhere else, but acceptance and respect in Britain were and to a large extent still are predicated on a class system. Although none of my family or friends, despite their class consciousness, ever made Robbie an outsider, the United States is more of a melting pot. Long before I thought of leaving Britain for professional reasons, I would look at my family, with its two fair-skinned and two darker people, and think, *America is the place for us*.

If either of our sons someday wants to make contact with his birth family, we will do everything we can to help—we still have some addresses and photographs to start the search. When Chris was still a baby, his natural grandmother sent him an egg cup and a silver spoon and a fabulous letter, forwarded to me by his foster family. She was still a young woman, in her forties at the time, and she had wanted to keep the baby herself, but her daughter didn't want that, and it could not be done without her permission. The daughter was obviously rebellious—the social workers intimated they were having a hard time with her—but the grandmother must have been a loving woman, and I hope some day she will see Chris again.

I've admitted that I'm not a spiritual person, and I don't think there is some all-knowing, all-powerful being directing the world order, or disorder. But there's a part of me that believes Robbie and Chris are the sons Andrew and I were "meant" to have. Robbie is the sensitive one, like his father—artistic, musical, poetic—and he seems to sail through life a little bit late for everything. Chris is a bomb, rushing and full of energy like me, and a control freak. It would not be possible to love them more if I had carried them in my womb—most of the time, I forget that I didn't, which is a common sentiment among adoptive parents. Andrew swears that my breasts grew bigger when we got Robbie, and bigger still with Christopher, like phantom pregnancy. Sometimes I look at Andrew's enviably thick head of black hair and think, *How nice— Robbie and Chris won't go bald*. And then: *Oh*. But it took some time for my own father to consider the boys his real progeny. His was an archaic way of thinking, probably not uncommon for men of his generation. (I knew that he would come to accept and adore them, and he did, becoming affectionate and generous with them both in life and in the bequests at his death in 1995.) But I was so in love with my children that no one else's passé notions of what constitutes a "bloodline" impinged on my happiness. I had my family.

# 9

IN THE SUMMER of 1985, Beatrix Miller announced her impending retirement from British *Vogue* after a twenty-year reign. We, her loyal minions, were devastated and felt insecure about the future, but we were also ambitious, and lots of people applied for the job, including me. Grace Coddington, the most senior person on staff, didn't really want to be editor, having no interest in all the job's many disparate obligations beyond the parameters of fashion. Although I was the executive fashion editor by then (I'd finally been made second in command to Grace), I didn't think I had a chance, because I had little grounding in features or production, but it felt like the right political gesture. Bernie Leser, the managing director of Condé Nast, was interviewing prospective candidates, and the joke was that you knew how you stood according to whether you were asked to interview in the A.M. or P.M. Dear Bernie liked a lovely long lunch and a little nap afterward, so the before-lunch bunch were the serious contenders. Naturally, I was scheduled for the afternoon. I rather timidly produced a cursory form of documentation about my qualifications for the job—I'd be ashamed of it today. At that time I had no real fire in the belly to be an editor-in-chief, no over-arching plan, and no substance beyond the demands of a fashion sitting. We had a nice chat that amounted to absolutely nothing.

By autumn we realized that the front-runner for Bea's job was Anna Wintour, creative director of American *Vogue*, who was getting restless under editor-in-chief Grace Mirabella. Anna, two years younger than me, was the daughter of a British newspaper editor and his American wife, and I'd known her since our days covering the lingerie market in the early 1970s. She went to the States in 1976 to work at *Harper's Bazaar*, the now defunct *Viva*, and *New York* magazine, but the savvy head of the Condé Nast empire, S. I. Newhouse, had marked her out as a rising talent and, amid much gossip, her ascension at British *Vogue* was announced.

A few months later, in the spring of 1986, Anna was ensconced in a small but chic house in Edwardes Square that faced a private garden bordered by black iron railings, meeting with the senior staff and, in particular, Grace Coddington, who was to continue as fashion director. Anna already had a reputation—it was said that she had had labor induced for the birth of her first child so she'd be ready to attend the couture collections. She rarely took off the dark glasses that camouflaged the thickness of her lenses; the effect was intimidating. (Even if there was a power failure at a fashion show, Anna would still sit there in the dark behind her shades.) We both got our blunt haircuts from a quirky fellow at the Michaeljohn salon named Charlie Chan, who was known for reading horoscopes and other New Agey amusements while he was snipping bangs, but it was reported that Anna told him to shut up. One of the first calls I got from her was to ask where she could store her furs. I had to conceal my bemusement: No one I knew in London wore furs, and *I* certainly couldn't afford them.

It was obvious we were heading for a direct culture clash: While Anna may be half-British by birth, she is thoroughly American in outlook. She was civilized and polite and reassuring about wanting us to stay on, but our fashion dreamworld had nothing to do with the sort of lifestyle she wanted to project in the magazine. Her meetings and memos made it clear that she was going to shake up British *Vogue*, make it faster and busier, directly addressing the concept of the modern working woman, and it scared the hell out of us. She hated anything contrived, unreal, overdone, wacky, ponderous, or too archly British. Gone were the Wellington boots and sittings at castles in the country. In came the briefcases and sittings at Lloyd's of London. Anna wanted nothing of the rocks-and-rubber work I'd been doing. She wanted smiling, happy, athletic, professional pictures. She wanted saneness and sameness. It was the end of life as we knew it.

There was a farewell cocktail party at Bea's house in Chelsea, which was like a page out of an elegant British shelter magazine, all chintz and mahogany and books lining the walls. But on her last day, I found Bea in her office at five o'clock and realized no one had organized a final goodbye—she was just going to walk out of there forever, alone, on a Friday night. I rushed down the street to a liquor store for champagne and got everyone together for a proper send-off. The decorators moved in over the weekend, painting the walls of Bea's office linen white, knocking down one wall to make a new entrance, setting in place an antique desk and Biedermeier sofa. Bookshelves were installed for bound back issues of the magazine and a large NO SMOKING sign was propped in the middle of them. The carpet was pulled up and the bare floors polished. And that was that: the changing of the guard.

For her first London collections, Anna was accompanied by André Leon Talley. André is a six-foot-seven black Southerner who tends to dress in riotous excess—striped stretch pants and red snakeskin backpacks, patent leather pumps with grosgrain bows, faux-fur muffs—and who had been, among other things, a receptionist at Andy Warhol's *Interview* magazine. We couldn't figure out whether Anna was planning to hire him, and if so, as what. Surely his personal style wasn't what she had in mind as a fashion imperative? (In fact, André never joined British *Vogue*, though he worked for Anna subsequently in New York.) We were all a bit thrown: She seemed to detest the outré—she had run out of the first Galliano show she ever saw, with its Captain Hook aesthetic—

134

and she was horrified at the sort of work I was doing, the icono-clastic images that differentiated British fashion coverage from anything in American magazines. I know this because, five years later, she wrote me a note about it, for a book of anecdotes and congratulations the staff made to commemorate my twentieth year at the magazine. "On my first day as editor-in-chief at British *Vogue*," she wrote, "Liz Tilberis, then executive fashion editor, proudly showed me some black and white photographs of young women wrapped up in head bandages, looking as if they'd dropped from Mars. 'This is very new!' she said. 'Oh, my God, I'm back in England,' I replied."

Salaries at British *Vogue* were abysmally low, but Anna demanded and got a reasonable, more American-style pay scale for us. When I went to New York for the collections in 1986, she called me from London and informed me I'd be getting a significant raise, from 23,000 pounds to 27,000. This was most unexpected.

"I don't know what to say," I sputtered.

"You could say 'Thank you,'" she retorted.

I've been accused of being too polite myself, to the degree that nobody knows what I'm talking about—if I want to kill an article, I tend to say, "Why don't we put that aside for a while?" instead of "I *hate* it!" Anna was the opposite extreme—peremptory and rather tactless, unconcerned with "the little people." She was quickly bored, very focused, and didn't let anything so mundane as courtesy get in her way. When she joined us in New York for the shows, I began to wonder how long I'd last and whether it was worth the angst. Anna and Grace started to argue about what clothes to shoot. Their first spat was over a double-layered coat by Ralph Lauren. The Algonquin Hotel faces south, and it was a bright day, with sunlight streaming onto the work table in the suite, but the mood grew black and combative.

"It's fabulous," said Grace. "We must include it."

"It's ridiculous," said Anna. "Why would you wear two coats?"

"It's the look," said Grace.

"But it doesn't make sense," said Anna.

It was the epitome of their classic dilemma: Grace was always going for the look, and Anna was always for the reader. I couldn't respond, take sides, break the tie—it was nothing to do with me. I was always ready to try something daring and provocative, but I am also nonconfrontational, and I suddenly felt I couldn't breathe—or cope. Panicked and gasping, I said, "I'm sorry, I've got to leave the room." It turned out that the tension had brought on asthma, and I was to suffer from it for years, going from hospital to hospital for tests, and eventually controlling it with a Swedish inhaler. (Chemotherapy finally wiped it out, and I've heard other cancer patients report that chemo cleared up their allergies. For the first time, I was able to stop coughing long enough to read a children's story aloud or attend a movie without being a public nuisance.)

Anna was adamant that fashion should be seen on the pages in a clear and instructive way. There was endless reshooting—if she didn't like it, it got done again and again. Grace's first sitting for her, featuring Yasmin Le Bon in an orange Jean Muir coat, had to be done three times until she got it right—with Yasmin holding tulips, running for a taxi. Anna wanted motion, models in the streets, looking as if they were off to work. Even though she was dictatorial, we were called in at every second to be part of the making of the magazine. Bea Miller had edited by osmosis and diffusion, working a kind of alchemy as she moved pages around on her office floor, protecting us from tawdry considerations of budget, page counts, advertising, copy flow. Anna didn't feel for one moment that we needed protecting. The fashion meetings were horribly tense. Every week we'd have a planning session to come up with stories for the next issue, the whole department talking about new clothes, new designers, new models. Anna, behind her sunglasses, would sit on a hard little chair and if she didn't appreciate an idea, she would tap her pencil loudly on the desk, and I'd have another asthma attack.

Grace suffered the most. Her habitual tardiness did not endear her to Anna. Once when Grace was late returning from lunch, Anna called her at San Lorenzo restaurant and ordered her back to the office at once. Anna wanted to impose her own specific vision on the clothes—fair enough, but Grace had been in charge of the fashion content at *Vogue* for nearly twenty years. It got so bad that Grace would have to go out onto the London streets with the crew in a van, set up a shot, then take a Polaroid picture and send it back to Anna at the office by messenger. Then Anna would call her in the van and say "Like it" or "Don't like it."

It was a steep learning curve for me too. On the morning of my father-in-law's funeral in November, Anna called me at home to tell me that the trip I was preparing to New York was over budget.

"You cannot take your assistant," she announced in a clipped voice. "It's far too expensive. Hire somebody when you get there." I was horrified to be reprimanded like a willful child, and I was hardly alone. There was a lot of complaining done by all as Anna tried to marshal an inherited team. She brought in a troika of her own people: personal assistant Gabé Doppelt, design director Michael Roberts, and features editor Emma Soames, the Churchill granddaughter who'd worked at British *Vogue* years before.

The word went out that we were a dysfunctional family, and a jewelry designer named Tom Binns made a pin that read "Vague Vogue Vomit." The British newspapers were dying to know what was going on in the bastion of high fashion, a place that had been a silent, impenetrable enclave for so many years. Beatrix Miller had loathed seeing her name in the papers and had done everything to avoid publicity. But Anna was high-profile, a perfect target for poisonous gossip. The press found it immensely entertaining that the "Voguettes," the dilettante daughters of the rich, were getting kicked into shape by a strict, slick Americanized import and started referring to Anna as "Nuclear Wintour" and "The Wintour of Our Discontent." The *Evening Standard* reported "her habit of crashing through editorships as though they were brick walls, leaving behind a ragged hole and a whiff of Chanel." She never reacted to any of this in front of the staff, and we were left to wonder how such savage and invidious press affected her.

Since Anna was thin and had great legs, she was accused when she took over British *Vogue* in 1986 of foisting the return of the mini on a less genetically endowed public. (In one episode of the British TV satire that came later, *Absolutely Fabulous*, the fashion-editor character named Patsy says, "One snap of my fingers, and I can raise hemlines so high that the world is your gynecologist.") The predilection for short skirts was already apparent at the Paris collections that season, but in fall of 1986, Anna was marginally ahead of most designers in judging that the mini's moment had arrived. Clothes that had been borrowed for sittings were returned to infuriated designers with six inches lopped off—in New York I had the tailor at the Algonquin cut down a coat. When hemlines change, every proportion is affected. Designers cannot tinker— they have to start from scratch. It's a myth that fashion is completely reinvented each season—it mostly evolves slowly with a different color palette, a new silhouette. Anna's takeover at British Vogue occurred at one of those rare moments of dramatic shift.

The mandate of a fashion magazine is to present a trend in an authoritative manner, to announce and then anoint a new theme. Anna was seen to be setting the pace. The carping about her may have been initiated by British designers who were reluctant to change and resented going along with a look that was perceived as more starkly modern and American than the typically dreamy and nostalgic English style. Eventually, the whole international fashion world ratified the short-skirted, big-shouldered business suit as the look of the mid-1980s. Soon everyone from fashion editors to corporate vice-presidents owned a padded-shouldered red-jacketed power suit with a short skirt, and we were all running to catch taxis in our black opaque tights and high-heeled pumps.

There was another cataclysmic shift closer to home. Just before Christmas 1986, Grace punctured my holiday spirit by announcing that she was leaving British *Vogue*. Her power struggle with Anna had worsened—Anna was demanding that new photographers be found, and Grace didn't like the dictates from on high. "You don't need a fashion director," she told Anna when she quit, "because you're it." Grace had been doing extracurricular work styling Calvin Klein's advertising campaigns, and she accepted a job as his design director in New York.

My first reaction was to burst into tears. Then I realized I had to pull myself together. I was next in line to inherit Grace's title of fashion director, but Anna and I had never squared our disparate views of fashion photography. I was still fighting her clear directive to make the clothes wearable, the models cheerful, the themes accessible. I liked my edge and never let her forget that I had been in the royal court of Queen Bea, and that I felt the new reign of mediocrity would never make such fashion nistory. But that didn't stop me from asking for Grace's position. Anna sidelined my request. Then one day she took me to lunch at the Westbury Hotel.

"You have to stop complaining," she said. "I'm tired of hearing about the good old, bad old days. You know how to do what I want—the question is, will you? If you want to stay, then back me up." I was angry and nervous, like a cornered animal, but I knew she was right. I wouldn't stand for any subversives on my team if I were in charge, and the pragmatic side of me wouldn't jeopardize my career. I never became a convert to Anna's themes and schemes, but I decided right then to be a dutiful number two.

In January 1987, I became fashion director. I had moved just about an inch up the masthead during my career at *Vogue*, but that inch meant I'd replaced the woman who was my idol when I started out. It didn't mean power or a fancy office—I just moved into Grace's glass cubicle in the fashion department, and instead of carrying out her bidding, I carried out Anna's bidding directly. It didn't mean that famous people took my phone calls, or that I got to fly first class, or that I earned gobs of money. It was a title of recognition for years of service. And I felt that Anna began to loosen up slightly and trust me—perhaps because I finally understood and delivered the kind of work she wanted, which was all about action and speed and up-ness, perhaps because she herself had conferred my title, so I now represented her own good judgment.

The Tilberises had outgrown the hand-me-down apartment from Andrew's parents and moved about a half mile away to our first house, a narrow brick townhouse with a lovely garden out back, a family with young children on the left, and a friendly elderly couple on the right. My parents would come for Sunday lunch, or we'd spend the weekend at their house in Bath. Andrew stayed home with Chris during the week, and I'd take Robbie to school in the morning, then do a U-turn in the worst rush-hour traffic on Regent Street, still terrified of being late for work, despite my promotion.

One day that spring, I was standing in my kitchen when the phone rang and an American voice said, "Hi, Liz, this is Ralph Lauren. Are you coming to the New York collections?" I said yes. "Can I meet you for breakfast on April first at the Plaza Hotel?" he asked. I said that I'd be delighted and put the phone down. Then I started getting paranoid. He had said April 1. Maybe it was just one of my friends playing a terrible joke on me.

To my relief, Ralph did appear on the appointed day and didn't take long to get down to business. "I wonder if you'd be interested in working for me," he said. The offer was completely unexpected, but not at all unwelcome. Ralph thought that an ongoing dialogue between a designer and a journalist could be effective. After my years at a magazine, I'd have useful ideas and opinions about advertising, about runway shows, about whether it was a moment for stripes or knits, for tight or baggy. But I wasn't sure I was ready to leave the relative glamour and prestige of fashion journalism for the grittier commercial world of Seventh Avenue, and said I would have to consider it. From the ladies' room in the hotel lobby, I called Grace at Calvin Klein, swearing her to secrecy. She expressed a hesitant enthusiasm for the idea but was strangely quiet. By the time I got back to my hotel room, there was a message from Calvin himself.

"What would you think about coming to work for me?" he asked.

My head was spinning. I'd never been a hot property. "I'd love to talk about it," I replied, "but I have this offer from Ralph."

"So come talk," he said. The next day, I went to Calvin's Seventh Avenue showroom. Over coffee, he explained that he was starting a moderately priced line called Classifications, a sporty American version of the budget *Vogue* fashion pages called "More Dash Than Cash," from his description. I would be the creative director of the line, a position similar to but more specific than the job at Ralph Lauren, and the salary would be enormous.

I was reeling. The figure was about five times what I was earning at British *Vogue*. I said I needed time to consider the offer and called my husband. Andrew had always been interested in going to America. He was an American history buff and had a real simpatico for the culture that produced jazz and blues—in fact, one of his first acts as a U.S. resident was attending a memorial service for Dizzy Gillespie. Above all, the idea of that much money sounded like winning the lottery. "I'll back you whatever you decide," he said, "but if both offers are bona fide, think about what it means to be working for Grace."

Two days later Ralph Lauren called again. "Are you frightened of helicopters?" he asked. "If not, would you like to come out to my house at Montauk on Friday to talk?"

I took a deep breath. "Actually," I said, "there's been a new development since we spoke. Calvin Klein has asked if I'd come on board there, and he's offered me a six-figure salary."

Ralph was clearly nonplussed. It *was* an extraordinary amount of money. He sort of cleared his throat and said, "Well, the offer to come out and talk still stands."

So I went to the heliport on the East River and boarded his private helicopter for a noisy thirty-minute ride to the easternmost point of Long Island, amazed at how many homes had swimming pools. I'd tried to dress Lauren-esque in linens and white plimsolls, the sneakers with a stripe like the mark on the hull of a merchant ship, but when I got out of the chopper at Montauk Airport, I stepped immediately into a puddle. Ralph's English butler met me and drove me to his beachfront house—not the English manor house I associated with his advertising, but a spare and low-ceilinged building, rather like a Japanese lodge, with a golf course-size lawn leading to the Atlantic and ebony irises planted around a freeform black pool. A salad was served on an L-shaped banquette in the dining room, and I nearly bit the inside of my mouth with what I had decided to say.

"In order to leave England, uproot the family, and put my boys

141

in school here," I said, "I really would need the exact amount Calvin has offered." He got a careful look on his face, not unfriendly but unsettled, and said he'd think about it. After polite conversation, we kissed goodbye. I flew back to the Fifty-ninth Street heliport, then to Kennedy Airport and straight on to London that night, my stomach in knots.

The fact that Ralph Lauren and Calvin Klein were interested in hiring fashion editors was a sign of the fast pace and international scope of the industry in the mid-1980s. The two men were already established as the world's foremost fashion marketers. Their acumen about advertising imagery and the absolute precision in defining brand identity was, and is, unparalleled. They liked what we were doing at British *Vogue*, our burgeoning connection with American photographers and locations, and they liked how we represented their clothes on our pages. We were able to impart or imply a distinct kind of lifestyle, and that's what they were selling, not just the clothes. Fashion is never just the clothes. It's about the appropriation of an image. Calvin Klein is about luxury so streamlined and self-assured, it could be sweet simplicity, and Ralph Lauren is tastefully preppy, an ode to the lifestyle of an English country house.

Back in London, after many more transatlantic conversations, I received an offer from Ralph matching the salary Calvin offered. I now had two equally dazzling deals on the table, but I realized I wanted to be on my own, rather than continuing to work in Grace's shadow. When I called Ralph Lauren to accept his offer, I was told he didn't do contracts. I wasn't about to pack up my family and my life on a handshake agreement, and when Andrew entered the conversation, he managed to convince Lauren's senior management to put the deal in writing. Then I called Calvin Klein to explain. He did not let sentiment affect his business sense. "You can't see my resort collections," he said, "because you're going to work for the competition." It was my first inkling of how my footing in the fashion world would change completely, how cut off I would be, no longer welcome in any showroom. But I'd been at British *Vogue* since I was twenty-one, and that September I was going to be forty. I thought I'd reached the ceiling of my career in London, and now that we had an opportunity for a new life in America, we were going to take it. We put our house up for sale and started packing.

Anna Wintour was pregnant with her second child, and her husband, a psychiatrist named David Schaffer, was commuting from New York. When I went into her office to resign in June 1987, I was fully aware of the rumors that she was lonely, hated seeing herself vilified in the British press, and hoped to go back to America herself. She looked at me incredulously. "Why didn't you tell me?" she exclaimed. "That's ridiculous. Don't you realize you won't be able to change one shirt button at Ralph Lauren?" Even though I was not being hired as a designer, her warning conveyed that I wouldn't be exercising much creative control, just carrying out the wishes of the man in charge. Her disparagement made my new job sound even less appealing than my current situation, carrying out *her* vision. But who could argue with a quarter of a million dollars? The British press announced that I was following in Grace Coddington's footsteps on my way to America, and my friends organized a going-away party at the Savoy Hotel. Two days later, Anna called me into her office and closed the door. "I'm leaving," she said. "Do you want to be the editor?"

I was completely and utterly thrown, shocked, stunned. Editing British *Vogue* was beyond anything I'd thought of for myself. It had always been my goal to be the best sittings editor possible, to produce wonderful pictures of beautiful clothes, and I'd achieved that. The responsibilities of an editor-in-chief go far beyond those self-contained parameters. She must have a strategic vision, a command of production schedules, insights about every arena of the magazine: features, arts, personalities, food, travel, health—not to mention the business side of the business: advertising, sales, and profitability. Different editors edit differently, but ultimately decisions about every subject, layout, title, photograph, and illustration rest on her shoulders. I was number two, but it was a tremendous leap to being number one. But with all that had happened in the intervening eighteen months, I had begun to see my capabilities in a new light.

I said yes on the spot. It was that irresistible a challenge. In a trance, I went down to see Richard Hill, managing director of Condé Nast's British operations, to explain that I wanted this job, but Andrew had to agree. We were packed and ready to leave for New York. If we were to do an about-face, the company would have to be financially persuasive. I called my assistant to get my car (a white Mini) and drive me around the block, circling Hanover Square again and again, until I calmed down enough to tell her what happened, swearing her to confidentiality. I had to tell someone, and I still didn't know how I was going to tell Andrew.

His reaction was just as I'd expected. "No!" he yelled. "Fuck it! The house is sold, our possessions are in cartons at the airport, and we're going." Then he must have seen the expression on my face—pleading and pathetic, perhaps, or dashed and desolate. "Do you really want this?" he asked. I nodded mutely. He squared his shoulders and said, "Okay, we'll stay, but on one condition: I go up there and negotiate with them. They'll have to pay for the undoing of our plans: a house, a car, a clothes allowance, the lot. No more child's play."

So Andrew acted as my agent. He had absolutely no experience in such matters, no training as a manager or lawyer or accountant. He just had enough bravado to go into Vogue House and thrash out a contract for more money than I could imagine. But one of *Vogue*'s conditions was non-negotiable: Since I had no experience with features, I had to accept the title of editor under Mark Boxer, who would become editor-in-chief. Mark was a highly respected figure in the British media establishment. He published biting serial cartoons under the byline "Marc" and had art-directed *Queen* magazine under Beatrix Miller in the 1960s, and the U.K. *Sunday Times Magazine* during its investigative heyday in the 1970s. First joining Condé Nast as editor of the humorously bitchy *Tatler* magazine, he had become editorial director of the company while Anna was at British *Vogue*, although his name was never above hers on the masthead. But his journalistic credentials were so strong, I had no choice but to agree.

With my new contract in hand, I had to pick up the phone and break the news to Ralph Lauren, backing out of a job at the last minute after he'd done everything to entice and accommodate me. But he was the perfect gentleman. He understood my professional dilemma and was gracious enough to congratulate me. I had to ask him to keep my confidence—Anna Wintour's move to New York was still top-secret, although rumors were flying. At the resort collections in July, I was spotted at Calvin Klein's show by Bernadine Morris, the canny fashion reporter of the *New York Times*. She instantly figured it out: If I wasn't banned from Calvin Klein, that meant I couldn't be going to work for Ralph Lauren, and *that* meant I must be staying where I was. But why? And what did it mean for Anna?

I fled town for Long Island and a sitting with Naomi Campbell wearing a Chanel couture Elizabethan gold-leafed pants outfit (her first British *Vogue* cover). *Women's Wear Daily* tracked me down at a local inn, but I had an assistant tell them, "Liz is on the beach." The calls and inquiries were incessant: What was happening to me, to Anna? I remained dumb and on the beach. The news broke in July when Louis Oliver Gropp, the editor-in-chief of *House and Garden*, got a call while he was at the beach, informing him that his magazine would henceforth have a new name, *HG*, and a new editor-in-chief, Anna Wintour, the latter to be replaced at British *Vogue* by one very nervous, excited, and unknown Elizabeth Tilberis.

# 10

IF MY HAIR hadn't already been gray, it would have changed overnight. The announcement of Anna Wintour's departure was a much bigger deal than my promotion, mostly because of speculation that *HG* was a mere pit stop in the Grand Prix of her career, with the finishing line at American *Vogue*. (We'd heard the story, perhaps apocryphal, that Grace Mirabella, the incumbent editor at *Vogue*, once asked Anna, then her creative director, what she wanted, and Anna replied, "Grace, of course I want your job.") I was a bit annoyed that Mark Boxer got most of the press attention on our side of the Atlantic, but I was a nobody, while he was a media darling—he knew every editor in Fleet Street, he was urbane and handsome, and he was married to a glamorous Armani-clad newscaster named Anna Ford (who didn't have a high regard for me—she used to call and ask me to recommend hairdressers).

It always boosts the esprit de corps when someone is promoted from within, rather than overlooked in a search for new blood, and the staff seemed pleased with my good fortune—except for one of the fashion editors, Anna Harvey, who sat in her office and cried because she'd wanted the job herself. Instead, she got a job as a creative consultant at Harrods, but an article in the London *Times* insinuated that she'd been hired to teach the new Egyptian owner, Mohamed al-Fayed, how to use a knife and fork at swank dinner parties. Fayed, who is in fact an elegant and debonair man, also owned the Ritz Hotel in Paris and resided in the Bois de Boulogne villa where the Duke and Duchess of Windsor had lived out their exile, as most of the world learned in the aftermath of Fayed's son Dodi's romance with the Princess of Wales. Mr. Fayed once gave us permission to do a couture sitting at the villa, where the duchess's shoes were still lined up in her closet. When the article appeared, Anna Harvey was summarily un-hired from Harrods and came back to work at British *Vogue*, so constructively that I (and the Princess of Wales) lobbied, unsuccessfully, for her to be editor when I left.

Generally when a new editor takes over at a magazine, the transition should be seamless for the reader, but I wanted to make my own statement with more cutting-edge clothes and smarter fashion writing—real explication about how things were changing and what the reader should do about it. Anna Wintour took me to lunch at the Connaught, the sumptuous old-fashioned hotel in Mayfair, to officially hand over the reins and talk about the staff. She'd just returned from maternity leave after the birth of her second child and was back in form, both professionally and physically, within three weeks. She was wearing one of the perfect little Chanel suits that were her uniform, and I was wearing what I always wore at the time: a pair of easy trousers and a linen shirt (crinkled, at that). Suddenly it dawned on me: I was going to be the editor of British *Vogue*, and I didn't have anything to wear.

The editor of a fashion authority is a hydra-headed monster who must woo advertisers, placate retailers, stroke photographers, salute established designers, nurture new ones, and act as an emissary of the magazine. While fashion editors who held the studio equivalent of a desk job could opt for an old-fashioned or eccentric style, the person at the top was supposed to look the part. I loved the clothes I photographed and was always squirreling away enough money for a garment that I coveted, but I didn't have the budget of the grandees on staff, and a designer's discount only went so far. However, with the most prudent application of discretionary income, I had acquired some elegant simplicity for evenings and parties—white silk shirts and black pants—but I didn't have good office clothes.

Now I was prepared to spend money, but in return I wanted to look as sleek and pulled together as possible on my size 12 frame. When one is other than skinny, it's important for clothes to have structure, and I called Catherine Walker, the French-born couturier who often dressed the Princess of Wales, to give me a strong and flattering silhouette. Arriving at her Chelsea Design Company, I took off my shoes and walked on ivory carpets in stockinged feet as she sketched and showed me fabrics. The first time I put on one of her jackets that had appeared on the cover of *Vogue*, I felt the beauty of perfectly tailored, well-fitted clothes—a powerful shoulder, a shaped waist, a sleeve that didn't migrate. I had a dozen others made over the years. My uniform consisted of a collarless jacket worn with big pearls at the neck, a slim skirt and black hose (which really do make the legs look thinner), carrying my papers in a navy quilted leather bag from Fendi.

Before Anna Wintour left, she did me the kindness of calling Karl Lagerfeld to say, "Take care of Liz." (With some chagrin, she later lamented that his caretaking has been rather too good.) Handwritten faxes started arriving, and they've never stopped, providing invaluable advice and insights into fashion and fashion-able people—about new models, about keeping couture modern, about historical references in his work, about the evolution of glamour and elegance. The Lagerfeld atelier is the nerve center of Paris fashion. Never has any man been so connected—to royalty, photographers, models, artists, clubgoers, everyone who makes the fashion world spin on its axis—and he always says, "I've been around a *long* time," implying he knows where the bodies are buried. He is wonderfully witty and also very wise about the business—for example, his theory about the appeal of young models: "You can only sell clothes *to* a forty-four-year-old woman when they're shown *on* a twenty-four-year-old woman." Once, during a season when none of the models seemed to have hips or thighs, he remarked, "The female shape doesn't work for mannequins anymore—I've had to order boy dummies."

Lagerfeld himself is known for his black Yohji Yamamoto suits, worn with a black camellia tiepin. (He once sent me some of the white powder he uses on his signature ponytail, but it got stopped in customs, mistaken for cocaine.) He is fluent in five languages, conversant with art, music, and opera, and employs a full-time librarian for his collection of 250,000 books, distributed among his various residences. Even behind the screen of the dark glasses he invariably wears and the fluttering fans he carries, he is beset by admirers, so he never goes to restaurants. A chef prepares sumptuous dinner parties at his eighteenth-century maison particulière in the middle of Paris, set on a massive lawn that seems to give off its own light, even at night. The gilded walls and eighteen-foot ceilings are set off by billowing purple silk drapes, and the dining table is laid with silver-and-vermeil cutlery made by the master silversmith Germaine—a spoon, Karl once said, would be the price of a car.

Although I knew which spoon and fork to use, it was dizzying to be included in his inner circle. *And* I acquired a lot of Chanel. Nothing equaled the feeling of going to the Chanel boutique in Paris, trying on the kind of perfectly constructed suit that seemed like second skin, and walking out onto the Rue Cambon with that suit wrapped in tissue printed with tiny *Cs* and tucked into the distinctive glossy black and white shopping bag. I actually felt taller. I was criticized for not being more visibly supportive of British designers, but every woman I knew was obsessed with the Chanel suit in all its many inventive manifestations—a scuba look one season, a denim trim the next, a medieval doublet after that—and when you're in fashion, you gotta have it. One of my big pleasures, after so many years of struggling with homemade and bargain-priced clothes, was to have a grown-up wardrobe. Designers want editors to be seen in their creations. It flatters them, gets them press coverage, and helps the branding of their name. When the name becomes synonymous with style, women who can't afford the clothes will still buy their mascara, their perfume, and their bed-sheets.

Dressed in Chanel by day, the moment I got home I changed into sweatshirts and leggings to take over from Andrew and our nanny, Jackie, cooking a supper of pasta or steak-and-kidney pie, reading a Beatrix Potter bedtime story, lamenting the loss of my lawn, which was appropriated for soccer games. I think that a good routine breeds confidence in children, and our boys had already had a complex start in life. I wanted them to feel secure in their little world. But there was scant danger of our family life falling victim to a more glamorous social schedule. Editors in Britain are not the media stars they are in America, not famous, not much noticed, not terribly important. I had a good job but not a bloated ego. And Andrew never got confused by my new status or paycheck. "If you get the sack tomorrow," he'd remind me, "half the people you think of as friends won't take your call."

My first day as editor was my fortieth birthday. When I walked into my office (Bea's office, as I thought of it, but still decorated by Anna), I found two desks, one for me and one for Mark Boxer, an inauspicious start. As my first editorial decision, I went into the art department and retrieved a photograph by David Bailey of Christy Turlington in a décolleté Calvin Klein shirt. Anna had killed it, but I loved it and wanted it for my first cover. The art director, John Hind, and I worked on the color for the logo, a gunmetal gray that harmonized perfectly with the cream of the clothing. Thrilled with the prospect of such a beautiful debut, I went home for a birthday dinner with Andrew and the boys—takeout fish and chips, wrapped in newspaper and washed down with champagne.

The next day, the logo was red.

"Mark came in and changed it," said John sheepishly.

"Oh, no, he fucking doesn't," I fumed. I was incensed and confused. I was supposed to be the editor and, after twenty years at *Vogue*, felt far more qualified to make visual judgments than Mark. I would have been glad for his input about features, but he had such weird, esoteric ideas. "Let's do a piece about the comeback of God," he'd say. I'd sit in meetings with his pretentious feature ideas about "the philosophy of greenery" or a profile of the chairman of the British rail system going right over my head, and the minute he left, I tried to make the story more reader-friendly.

It's impossible to have two people in charge of editorial policy and decisions. We clashed constantly, not even so much about substance as about management style. I edit by encouragement and discussion. Mark was much more autonomous and brusque. He was a dictator, and I was an oligarchist. "Don't be an idiot," he'd bark at someone, and I'd have to deal with the repercussions from a bruised staff. He rode a black motorcycle, and if I saw it in the garage when I arrived in the morning, I knew it was going to be a difficult day. But only a few months into our partnership, Mark became jaundiced and began to suffer from headaches. Before anyone knew what was happening, he was in the hospital, diagnosed with an inoperable brain tumor. He continued to work from home for a while, and I'd take him layouts, keeping him involved at least in spirit, all of his bark and bite gone. When he died at age fifty-seven in the summer of 1988, I was genuinely sad. He was a talented man, but the two of us had been locked in an impossible bloodless fray. A year later, when I was finally given the title of editor-in-chief, it felt like a hollow victory.

With Mark gone, I found a strong features editor in Alexandra Shulman, whom he'd initially terrorized at *Tatler*, screaming, "How can you be so boring and predictable?" and sent crying to the bathroom. In fact, she was good enough to get poached for the editorship of British *GQ*, after eighteen months at *Vogue*, and I promoted her deputy, Eve MacSweeney. I wanted to address the intellectual pursuits of a woman who's interested in fashion, to introduce a mix of analytical journalism and sharp reporting on the culture. Despite my derision of Mark Boxer's intellectual pretensions, I wanted my features to be more highbrow than they were under Anna's regime: An excerpt from a novel had to be literary. Instead of interior decoration, we'd do architecture. And I wanted the strongest possible health articles: childhood depression, the aftermath of violent crime, Germaine Greer facing

151

menopause, men in the delivery room. Not surprisingly, one of the first features I commissioned was about adoption. We also looked at the contemporary love poem, private versus state schooling, the British antipathy toward modern anything, the background of the Nobel Prize. (Alfred Nobel's wife was said to have absconded with a mathematics professor, which may explain why there is no Nobel Prize in math.)

I wanted to give readers something they'd not read in other British magazines: *Harpers & Queen* had a snobbish sort of elegance, and *Tatler* was gossip-driven. The hardest part was celebrity profiles—Britain is such a small market that Hollywood isn't that interested in being covered in our magazines. We had to take what we could get and then put up with major ego in a minor star. Janet Jackson even sued us. We'd gone to great expense shipping couture dresses to her in Los Angeles, and to justify the cost, we decided to do a cover try. But she assumed it was a done deal. Eventually, an arrangement was worked out and more pictures were taken, though she never graced the cover of British *Vogue*.

In the fashion pages, I wanted a return to glamour. Anna liked the normal, and I like the cutting edge. I felt what was lacking was the element of fantasy—the fancier, flashier, sometimes trashier, more extravagant, and even eccentric clothes. I raided the *Observer* newspaper to hire Sarah Mower as a fashion writer. Sarah brought clarity and gravitas to a subject as frivolous as hemlines and examined the fashion world's infinitely changing personalities, who were often more interesting than movie stars. I promoted a volatile, voluble blonde named Sarajane Hoare as fashion editor. She'd been languishing doing the "Men in *Vogue*" pages. Under her stewardship, the most imaginative photographers produced the most powerful images. Steven Meisel shot Isabella Rosellini and Tina Chow as circus stars in fishnets, gold bras, and leopard spots. Herb Ritts showed Brigitte Nielsen flexing oiled muscles in an evening gown. Peter Lindbergh had Linda Evangelista dressed as Guinevere, striding with greyhounds in Deauville. Patrick Demarchelier tracked Cindy Crawford strutting through the streets of New York City in swimsuits and stilettos. (There was a standard order in the art department in those bowdlerized days: Airbrush Cindy's mole.) These visual mythologies about medieval heroines, New Age goddesses, and red-hot dominatrixes reflected the soaring female ego of the late 1980s. Women were delighted to see themselves celebrated as powerful and commanding, in business and in bed.

The managing editor, Georgina Boosey, had been at *Vogue* since 1956 and had already nannied Anna Wintour through her infancy as editor. She did it again for me, quietly and discreetly teaching me about production, pagination, printing, and budgets. I didn't know that magazines had a house style of punctuation, that the size of text could be altered, that the fledgling issue got sent down to the printer in sections called forms and signatures. I had no idea how many words fit onto a page or what writers were paid. And I had to learn the balancing act of editorial against advertising. (My golden rule is that the solid "well" in the middle of the magazine is unbroken by advertising. It's like PBS, whereas the rest of the magazine is like commercial TV.) In my innocence I'd say, "We can put this here and that there," and Georgie would say, "I don't think so." Even more important, she had years of experience in the arenas of office politics and personnel. When ever there was a drama I needn't be pulled into—an assistant who wanted a promotion, an editor who took too much petty cash, a holiday schedule that left the office empty—she handled it.

Coming from a visual background, I felt quite at ease with John Hind, the art director for all my work under Bea Miller and Anna Wintour. The art department was a haven of whiteness and order compared to the mess of the fashion closet, and its inner sanctum was the projection room, with access granted only to senior staff. There John and I performed the time-honored ritual of viewing transparencies on a screen, reemerging like bats after hours of sitting in darkness with endless cups of tea. Then I'd put the reduced images of the pages, called "minis," up on my wall to monitor the pace and rhythm of each issue. Those were some of my happiest moments, the times when the mythic glamour of being the editor of *Vogue* felt most thrillingly real. Sometimes, if a picture was strong enough, we'd ignore all commercial wisdom and use it with a single coverline, unwilling to intrude on the beauty of the image with hard-selling text. Our record low was two words: Helena Christensen in a long white dress leading a white horse through the desert, against a background of bluest skies and the words "International Collections." That would be unthinkable now. Ten coverlines, three of which scream about sex, seem obligatory for most women's magazines these days, but ten years ago in the U.K., when the newsstands were less crowded, we got away with it.

It's only in retrospect that you understand the times you've lived through, but now I get it: Yes, I was lunching on sevruga at the Kaviar Kaspia and driving hell-for-leather in the new BMW negotiated by Andrew, with the limited-edition soundtrack from the Chanel runway show pumping through the car stereo. Yes, I was wearing designer clothes and my family moved to posher residences: first a brief sublet in Well Walk near the Hampstead Heath, where we lived opposite Boy George and regularly found teenage girls encamped on our lawn, then a lovely narrow brick Regency house in St. John's Wood, near the Beatles' Abbey Road and across the street from the Clifton Arms, the tavern where Lillie Langtry had assignations with her Prince of Wales.

But the real exhilaration of those years at British *Vogue* was that we were beholding the exact moment when fashion crossed over, transformed from a minority-interest subject into a front-page, prime-time obsession. In the free-spending 1980s, there was so much discretionary income that fashion reaped the rewards: Collections were making big and exotic statements, advertisers were buying lavish numbers of pages, and every main street of every major city was lined with designer boutiques, not to mention a Benetton in even the most remote Mediterranean village. High fashion reached the global community and suddenly fashion mattered to a lot more people. And we were witnesses, provocateurs, and recorders of this seismic shift.

The ultimate symbol of that late-1980s bonanza was the invention of the supermodel. Christy Turlington, Linda Evangelista, Naomi Campbell, and Cindy Crawford had begun their careers

154

when Anna Wintour was editing British *Vogue*, but they were babies then. By the end of the decade, they were in full command of their looks, experience, and sex appeal, turning these assets on to a degree that virtually scorched the camera. When talented photographers transferred the heat to the page, the designers began paying megabucks to put the models in their shows and advertising. And once TV cameras and newspaper photographers were given unprecedented access to the shows, millions of viewers and readers were clamoring to know who these women were, who they dated, what they ate for breakfast. They were more glamorous and enigmatic than most Hollywood actresses, and like the movie stars they were eclipsing, they had handlers and handmaidens. Early on in their careers, *Vogue* identified them in captions, breaking the convention of anonymity that had, with a few rare exceptions, ruled modeling until then, and suddenly they were household names. In making them personalities, we also contributed to the inflation of model fees exemplified in Linda Evangelista's tongue-in-cheek comment, "I don't get out of bed for less than ten thousand dollars a day."

Other famous "models" also required special handling. When we decided to do a portrait of the newly elected prime minister, John Major, and his wife in 1990, the photographer had to be somebody the Majors might have heard of, ergo Lord Snowdon. I supervised this sitting myself in the official home above the shop at No. 10 Downing Street. Alistair Jolly, the *Vogue* driver, and I were the stand-ins for the couple as Snowdon adjusted the lighting, but when the PM arrived home, Snowdon didn't like his choice of shirt.

"Can we get him to change his shirt?" I whispered to his wife.

"If I ask him, he'll be angry," said Norma Major. "*You* ask."

So I tiptoed upstairs with an armful of shirts from Savile Row and knocked on the prime minister's bedroom door.

"Excuse me, sir," I said meekly, "could you put on one of these?"

"Certainly," he said, and started to disrobe. It was an interesting moment: helping to dress the bare-chested leader of Great Britain in his bedroom. After the sitting, we were offered a glass of sherry, and the prime minister took us out to the garden. Just days before, the IRA had bazookaed a bomb over No. 10, trying to hit the Cabinet in session, but had succeeded only in blowing up a pear tree, and the prime minister proudly showed us the hole left in the garden wall.

I met the then prime minister again some months later, when I was invited by Prince Andrew and the Duchess of York to go to dinner at their new home on the edge of the Windsor Great Park. I was intrigued: the design and construction of the house had been a running gossip item in the English press, which dubbed it "South Fork," after the Ewing ranch in the hit soap opera *Dallas*.

The invitation did not extend to my husband, so I set off down the M4 with Alistair, the *Vogue* driver, and I don't know which one of us was more nervous as we entered the huge gates. The drive was long, with wooden fences on either side, and eventually the car drove between two large columns and into a walled court-yard. I walked up the wide steps and under the huge porch with circular supporting columns, to be welcomed by Prince Andrew himself.

The front doors opened into a very light wooden lobby with a high ceiling, which immediately made me think of a Swedish church. Candles and orchids were everywhere, and a large staircase led to the second floor, where a very young princess was obviously unhappy about going to sleep. The wails went on until the duchess herself, having said hello, bounded upstairs to settle down her daughter.

Prince Andrew walked with me into the huge rectangular drawing room. It was so large that it made the chairs and the fireplace look small. It was comfortable, rather formal, and extremely luxuriously furnished. The prince was obviously very proud of his new home. He gave me a short tour of the ground floor and received compliments with great pleasure.

Several people had already arrived and were standing talking near the fire. I already knew Lord and Lady Hesketh. He was at that time minister of trade, and his wife, Clare, who is very beautiful and terrific company, was a close friend of an editor at *Vogue*, who had introduced me to them. I did not know the Japanese ambassador and his wife, nor did I know political adviser Gordon Reese. When it was time to greet John Major and his wife, Norma, I joked about seeing him with his shirt off at our previous meeting. He looked rather shocked.

The best part of the evening was the end of the meal, when Prince Andrew asked the prime minister about the developing situation in Russia. Just days before, Mikhail Gorbachev had been on holiday at the Caspian Sea when Boris Yeltsin had assumed power in Moscow. The prime minister described how Gorbachev had been listening to the BBC World Service and heard the news of the takeover. He had immediately phoned John Major and asked what he knew. So there was a kind of hot line between the BBC, the Caspian Sea, and No. 10 Downing Street. Mr. Major had kept the unseated Russian premier abreast of all developements for the next twenty-four hours. There was something so magical about listening to him tell this piece of history to us all at that dinner table, I felt quite giddy being in such proximity to power.

Eventually the grown-ups left. Alexander Hesketh had said to me during dinner, "Hang on until the end because that's always such fun," and it was. Prince Andrew's descriptions of his life in the navy and of naval traditions were hilariously funny. I think we must have left well after midnight with the prince and the duchess standing on the steps of their lovely home waving until the last car had left the long drive.

Although such events were rare in my life, this was not my only dinner with a prime minister. Two years earlier, I attended a small dinner hosted by Lord and Lady McAlpine of Westgreen for the then prime minister Margaret Thatcher and her husband Denis. Alastair McAlpine was then the treasurer of the Conservative Party, and his vivacious wife, Romilly, was a friend of mine. Other guests included the actor Michael Crawford, Alan Yentob, who was head of BBC 1, and the playwright Ronald Harwood.

We dined in a cozy candlelit dining room in the McAlpines' small brick townhouse near the Houses of Parliament. Looking out the windows toward Westminster Abbey, I was a little nervous—this was a time of great IRA activity in London and there seemed to be a rather casual attitude to security. Being anywhere near Margaret Thatcher was a risk in itself.

Alistair and Romilly, who are world-class hosts, knew the prime minister well, and it was a very relaxed evening until at one point the conversation changed. I think the prime minister was waxing poetic to Michael Crawford about the plane-to-plane refueling of the fighter jets going to the Falklands. During a lull in her monologue, Ronald Harwood, who had been discussing the theater with Andrew, leaned across to ask her if she had seen "Breakthrough at Reykjavík," his television drama about the Reykjavík summit. She in turn leaned ominously over the table toward him and said that she wouldn't go to see it. Ronald asked why. "Because," she said, "it's *rubbish*!" He looked rather nonplussed and said, "But, Prime Minister, how do you know it's rubbish if you haven't seen it?" To which she replied, "It must be rubbish because you weren't there." The atmosphere had cooled considerably in the dining room and I thought Andrew was very brave when he parried her statement by saying, "If you can write about history only if you were there, that knocks out most history books, not to mention Shakespeare and the Bible!" But she waved at both men as if to try to make them vanish, and returned to her conversation about the Falklands. It was a very fierce moment.

I VAGUELY REMEMBER a day early in my career when I noticed a coltish sixteen-year-old sitting on a suitcase as she stopped in to visit her sisters at Vogue House on her way to boarding school. When nineteen-year-old Diana Spencer became engaged to the Prince of Wales, her vulnerability and nervousness were visible in the pictures British *Vogue* published. Because the magazine was so intertwined with the Spencers and the Windsors, it was easy and natural for the editors to help the new princess find a wardrobe for her daunting round of public duties. She decided to support the home team by wearing only British labels, and Anna Harvey was appointed as a kind of personal shopper for her, researching the market, calling in gowns she thought appropriate, and taking them to the princess's apartment at Kensington Palace for her perusal. If Diana had been naive about fashion before her royal induction, she proved a fast learner, confidently forming her own relationships with designers and becoming a fashion icon in the British press. Lots of us would love to take credit for her metamorphosis from dowdy schoolgirl to sexy sophisticate, but she really did it herself. Dominated by palace protocol during her marriage, she rarely spoke in public, and choosing her own outfits must have been one of the few ways she could assert her individuality and identity.

When I became editor, Anna Harvey introduced me to the princess, and periodically we'd have lunch at one of her stylish regular haunts, San Lorenzo or Le Caprice, where she would have her back to the room for privacy and her bodyguard sitting at the bar. It was an inherently odd and awkward situation, and initially I was inhibited about the conversation, but she was so disarming, I gradually felt at ease. Since our sons were about the same age, we had a commonality of interests and concerns. She often talked about her hopes for her sons to be equal to the demands that would be made of them, but also to be in touch with modern life and ordinary people. She felt she was waging two wars: against the antiquated protocol of royalty and against the tabloid press. She'd barter with the paparazzi: If she was traveling and staying at a hotel, she'd try to appease them by giving them one exit by the front door and the rest via the kitchen, knowing that if she tried to escape them altogether, they'd never leave her alone. At one point she met with Rupert Murdoch to ask for some consideration and privacy from his newspapers, but he offered no concessions.

In the fall of 1991, at a reception for the British Fashion Council Awards at the Royal College of Art, I introduced the princess to Linda Evangelista, who was emerging as the decade's über-model. That was a moment: two of the most beautiful, most famous, and most photographed young women in the world, coming face to face. At their urging, I arranged for the three of us to have coffee at a popular café called Joe's, owned by my friend Joseph Ettegdui, the owner of Joseph boutiques, who opened the restaurant especially for us but "cast" it with a few of his friends so it wouldn't look uncomfortably empty. In one of her regular transformations, Linda had just dyed her hair an attractive auburn, but the princess thought she was too thin. I had no idea that Diana had struggled with her own eating disorder and was sensitive to weight issues. I think she also felt a kinship with models and their subjection to endless scrutiny, fawning, and criticism.

British *Vogue* was traditionally viewed as the quasi-official documenter of the royal family, a patriotic privilege that had been most recently continued by Lord Snowdon, despite his divorce from Princess Margaret, and he had an affectionate relationship with Beatrix Miller. When he published a book of portraits titled *Sitting*, she sent him a fake cover made up by the art department, with a chicken hatching an egg. I once sent him out with an editor named Candida Lycett Green on a shoot featuring farm animals. A large pig had been shampooed and groomed, with glistening peach powder rubbed into its skin, but it wasn't happy and charged at Snowdon, knocking over the tripod and sending his assistant running for cover. Candida was delighted. She said she couldn't tell Snowdon what to do, but the pig could.

I realized that I had better start living up to *Vogue*'s tradition as court chronicler. Princess Diana's official portraits had always been so stiff and formal, hardly reflecting the relaxed modernity of the young woman I knew, and I had a vague idea that I'd like to do things differently. I wrote to her asking whether she'd consider being photographed with her sons and sent the letter over to Kensington Palace with the portfolios of three photographers: Bruce Weber, Alex Chatelain, and Patrick Demarchelier. Patrick's book included a *Vogue* cover with one of his young sons wrapped up in the model's shawl-collared coat. The princess liked it, and she liked Patrick, the consummate charming Frenchman—a big, bearish man with dark unruly hair and an accent so thick that, although he's lived in the United States for more than twenty years, television shows were known to use subtitles for his appearances.

(On an advertising shoot once, the client said to Patrick's assistant, "Could you please tell him I don't speak French?" The assistant looked pained and replied, "He's speaking English.")

The sitting took place at Highgrove in August 1989, the prince and princess's country house in Gloucestershire, which we thought would make a relaxed, informal background. Patrick decided to shoot in black and white, which is easier and more foolproof than color for great portraits, and he had to make sure it worked the first time, with no reshooting, given the time restraints set by the palace. The princess was wearing a white shirt, frolicking in the hay barn with William and Harry, a winning scene and a great coup for *Vogue*, but we weren't allowed to use the pictures on the cover. Buckingham Palace had the ultimate veto on the use of royal photographs, and the queen said no. I could only imagine that she thought a hay barn was not a regal enough image.

The second time Patrick and the princess teamed up, she was posed in the ultimate white satin ballgown and tiara, but instead of sitting ramrod straight in a chair, she was on the floor laughing with her head thrown back, the folds of the gown pooling around her. The photographs were breathtaking, radiant, glowing, and I desperately wanted one for the cover. The princess asked the queen herself. Again the answer came back: No. I didn't understand what was behind these refusals, still imagining that the unstuffy informality of the picture was deemed improper. As time has shown, the reasoning was probably more subtle. The photos represented one of the earliest public signs of the princess's growing determination to be her own person, and the palace was reining her in. Hugely disappointed, we did a cover mock-up of the photo with the prettiest sugar-pink British *Vogue* logo on it, and sent it over to the princess as a souvenir, receiving a gracious thank-you note in return.

Patrick had taken even more informal photographs of Diana wearing a black turtleneck and leggings, sprawled on the floor in an insouciant, slightly balletic pose. Our December 1991 issue was dedicated to dance, and I thought the image would be perfect for the cover, since the princess was a patron of the English National

Ballet. I put a call through to her private secretary, and Diana picked up the phone.

"Ma'am," I said, "there's the most fantastic cover here."

"Right," she said, "I'm coming over to see."

I alerted the staff, just to make sure no one would have a heart attack encountering her in the corridor, and when she arrived, everybody had their eyes studiously fixed on their work, as if the visitor were an insurance salesman. We showed her in to the projection room, and she chose the cover on the spot. It was one of those moments as an editor when you know you've got something so good, you get chills.

"So what happens now?" I asked.

"Just go ahead," she said, looking only slightly defiant. Buckingham Palace notwithstanding, the Princess of Wales was our stunning Christmas cover, which was reproduced in every newspaper in England. If there were any repercussions from the palace, I never heard about them.

I can't look at her photographs anymore, those glorious images of a most vibrant woman. The pictures Patrick Demarchelier took of the princess over a ten-year period—both for British *Vogue* and *Harper's Bazaar*—have been endlessly reproduced across the world since her death. The black-turtleneck sitting became the cover of *Newsweek* two days after Diana was killed, and the white-ballgown picture was placed in the window of Harrods as a memorial, alongside a photo of Dodi Fayed.

IT TURNED OUT that Anna Wintour *was* a lady-in-waiting. *HG* was a temporary dalliance for a woman destined to work in fashion—in fact, one witticism had it that the magazine was renamed for her tenure so people wouldn't call it *House and Garment*. Anna's real destination was American *Vogue*, where in July 1988, after less than a year at *HG*, she replaced Grace Mirabella as editor-in-chief. The latter, according to an oft-repeated tale, learned of her dismissal after it was announced on the evening news. Grace Mirabella herself had replaced the legendary Diana Vreeland, who had been given her walking papers in 1971, after nine years at the helm, by Alexander Liberman, the Soviet émigré who was editorial director of Condé Nast. The trenchant Vreeland later observed, "I have known White Russians; I have known Red Russians; I have never before known a yellow Russian."

Anna Wintour now had a power base befitting her desire to put her imprimatur on style, and in one of those ubiquitous little full circles, Grace Coddington became her creative director. At Calvin Klein, Grace had missed the action and tempo of doing sittings, and after living in America for a while, she understood the modern, working-woman, running-in-the-street, Americanized style Anna had been trying to impose at British *Vogue*. One Friday afternoon she called Anna and said, "I'd like to come back," and Anna, without missing a beat, said, "I'm starting on Monday. Why don't you start with me?"

I thought it was a terrific idea. We were all Voguettes once more, on both sides of the ocean, and I was on a professional high. London had not been the epicenter of fashion for a long time—we'd felt like the poor stepsister to Paris and Milan. But British *Vogue* was celebrating its seventy-fifth anniversary in June 1991 with a big cocktail party at the Royal College of Art, alma mater of some local young guns of fashion, showcasing photographs from the magazine over the years. We'd invited the world's top designers to make outfits with the word *Vogue* cunningly worked into knitwear, beadwork, or silkscreen, which we displayed on mannequins arranged on the staircase like a vision from a Busby Berkeley musical. When the acceptances started coming in, the guest list was an astonishing tribute from the fashion glitterati: Karl Lagerfeld, Gianni Versace, Azzedine Alaia, Gianfranco Ferré, Vivienne Westwood, Jasper Conran, and Valentino (whose date for the party was to be Joan Collins). I went to my publisher, Richard Shortway, with the list of acceptances; most of the guests were flying in from other parts of Europe or the States. He was so impressed that he took my hand and led me into the office of Richard Hill, the managing director of the company.

"Have you seen this list?" Shortway asked. "We have to feed these people!"

"Hmmph," said Hill with Condé Nast parsimony in his voice, "I suppose so." I was allowed to arrange a dinner at Mark's Club, a quintessentially British place with Highland scenes on dark red walls and meals that started with Scotch broth and ended with bread-and-butter pudding. It cost 8,000 pounds. We ate by candle-light, and the last of us had to be tossed out near dawn. I wore a jacket of pearls and bugle beads and a silver satin skirt designed by Catherine Walker especially for the occasion. It was the first time I ever gave a speech—short and sweet but a personal triumph. That dizzy, happy moment was the culmination of everything I had set out to achieve at British *Vogue*: The elite of the fashion community were honoring the magazine, and our circulation figures had climbed to an all-time high.

In my scrapbook is a poignant reminder of that party, an aerial shot of the entire staff on bleachers outside the Royal College of Art, looking up and laughing at the photographer Terence Donovan behind the camera, a massive, gesticulating figure hoisted a hundred feet in the air on a mobile crane. Terry was one of my dearest friends and closest confidants from my earliest days in fashion, part of a hugely talented and irreverent triumvirate, along with David Bailey and Brian Duffy, christened the "Terrible Three" by Cecil Beaton. All three had grown up in the rough-and-tumble East End of London (Terry never got over his glee at the idea of a truck driver's son owning a Rolls-Royce), and they produced the seminal fashion photography of the 1960s, replacing the serene and stately portraits of an earlier era with gritty, startling, unorthodox, and frankly sexual imagery. A 1964 article in the *Sunday Times* called them "The Modelmakers," and they reveled in their iniquitous reputations for shagging (British for screwing) their subjects.

My first memory of Terry is a Cockney voice booming from his sixth-floor studio in Covent Garden to his secretary in the base-ment: "Bridge to engine room!" From that moment on, I knew this man was going to be fun, often speaking in a private code that revealed his fascination with espionage. He'd call up and whisper,

"Alpha, Victor, Charlie, Delta, Tango," and then hang up, expecting me to decipher the invitation to lunch at one o'clock. Before he proposed to his wife, Diana, he had her handwriting analyzed, and the proposal itself was a letter bound in gold tape, announcing a wedding the following Thursday.

We did countless sittings together, trying to make something new out of a dead-on-arrival suit, trying to pump some chic into "More Dash Than Cash." But Terry's impact went far beyond fashion. One day in 1986 he called me with an offer. "Got a job, doll," he said. "Pop video. Robert Palmer. Not a big handbag, mind you." (This was code for a small budget.) I couldn't have cared less—I was thrilled at the opportunity. My job was to style six models who would be dancing in formation, rather zombielike, and pretending to play guitar as if they were band members. To fit with the lyrics, Terry wanted them sexy, and I chose identical tight black Azzedine Alaïa dresses. "Addicted to Love" turned out to be a seminal music video that made an indelible visual impression. Tom Ford, the designer for Gucci, told me that the sleek black leather looks of his 1997 "After the Fall" show were inspired by that video.

One afternoon in November 1996, Terry walked out of a sitting for British GQ, left his Silver Cloud parked on the street, and disappeared. Later that night a watchman found him hanging from the rafters in his West London painting studio. He'd been losing weight on diet pills, having painful dental work, and taking steroids for the eczema that was common among photographers who work with chemicals. An inquest revealed that the combination of medications must have caused a severe depression. Only weeks before, Andrew and I had flown to London for Terry's sixtieth birthday party, where he made a moving speech about courage, and his wife told me he'd been thinking of my fight against cancer, but none of the friends celebrating him that night, including fellow photographers David Bailey and Lord Snowdon, had a clue about Terry's own health or his state of mind. The mourners at his memorial service were a testament to his influence in so many areas of British life: former prime minister Margaret Thatcher, the

Princess of Wales, the Saatchi brothers of advertising fame, the Lords McAlpine and Palumbo, several generations of Condé Nasters, from the executives to the go-fers, his instructor from the local judo club he supported, and his East End childhood friends.

Terry had a soulful wisdom that made him an early convert to Buddhism, but he also had a wicked sense of humor, and a wonderfully mischievous approach to life. "Who cares about the pix?" he'd say about his visionary work. "It's all about crumpet" (crumpet being related to shagging). And he had a sixth sense about the times I needed to be encouraged or rescued: I'd hear him padding down the office hallway in the soft-soled black shoes that he found in Russia and wanted to import in one of his many business schemes, or I'd get a mysterious two-second phone call delivering a whispered command: "Five at the Italian"—Ciccone's restaurant, where he had a regular table. Often I'd escape the pressure and routine of the office for a bowl of pasta and a diverting anecdote. To ease the Princess of Wales through her first sitting with him, he held a 10-pound note in front of the lens and asked, "Recognize any relatives?"

The day Terry Donovan took that aerial photograph of the *Vogue* staff, I never imagined it would become a memento mori. It was intended as a token of his pleasure and participation in my success. When I came to America, we'd talk on the phone often. He loved what we'd done with *Harper's Bazaar*. "Laying out magazines is easy, doll," he'd say. "I could do it with my dick. And you've made it look as easy as it is." But that day in 1991 as we all sat for Terry, I thought my life couldn't get any better, that I had realized my most daring dreams and brazen ambitions, that I needed no other reward or challenge. I was wrong. As it turned out, the last months of 1991 were to be my last at British *Vogue*. It was getting to be time for me to leave.

166

# 11

THE FIRST MOMENT any notion of *Harper's Bazaar* came into my head was one glorious summer evening in 1991 on the rooftop of the Villa Medici in Rome, where 600 international guests were celebrating Valentino's thirty-year career at a party billed as "Trent'Anni di Magia." Even if you didn't speak Italian, you knew there was magic in the air. A circular stone staircase was lit by candles and flares, a gold-leafed cake was shaped like the designer's headquarters at Piazza Mignanelli, and dancers did the tarantella on the terrace for a succession of Rothschilds, Agnellis, and Von Furstenbergs wearing the couturier's most bejeweled creations, with Elizabeth Taylor outdazzling them all in plunging crystal-beaded chiffon and lace.

I was waiting in the buffet line when I saw Bernadine Morris of the *New York Times*, who had an inquisitive look on her face. "Liz," she said provocatively, "you know you're on the short list for the *Bazaar* job?" I just laughed. Technically, there was no *Bazaar* job. Anthony Mazzola, the magazine's editor of the past twenty years, was still at his desk. But *Bazaar* had slipped out of sight as a fashion force, and a shakeup was thought to be imminent. While it was flattering to be talked about as a potential editor of a venerable American magazine, I hadn't been approached about the job, nor was I looking for a job. I *had* a job, the sort of job that got me invited to Valentino parties. I went home and thought nothing more of it.

But the same gossip that was in the air on a Rome rooftop had been circulating in New York. Veronica Hearst, wife of Randolph Hearst, head of the family empire, was rumored to be lobbying for a new *Bazaar* editor, and even interviewing prospective candidates over tea at her fabulous Fifth Avenue apartment. The prospect of a corporate rumble loomed: Condé Nast (with its stable of *GQ*, the *New Yorker, Glamour, Vanity Fair, House and Garden*, and *Vogue*) and Hearst (with *Cosmopolitan, Good Housekeeping, House Beautiful, Town and Country, Redbook, Esquire*, and *Harper's Bazaar*) were rivals of long standing, historically pirating each other's personnel, but the only time Hearst had been able to challenge the supremacy of *Vogue* was the thirty-year reign of *Harper's Bazaar* under the legendary direction of Carmel Snow, Alexey Brodovitch, and Diana Vreeland, which had ended in 1962.

Carmel White Snow was born in Dublin but grew up in Chicago and New York after the death of her father, the managing director of the Irish Woolen Manufacturing and Export Company. (She and I shared an ancestral connection with the British textile industry, as well as our prematurely white hair.) The young Carmel assisted her mother in an exclusive dress shop called Fox and Company on Fifty-seventh Street, but when a fashion columnist for the *New York Times* helped her get an introduction at *Vogue*, she realized she wanted to report fashion, not sell it. An innovative fashion editor (a pet of Condé Nast himself and the only one with whom Edward Steichen would work), she didn't marry until age thirty-nine and had three daughters in her forties. In 1932, still hospitalized after the birth of her third child, she was approached by William Randolph Hearst to edit *Harper's Bazaar*, setting up an intense rivalry— *Vogue* personnel were forbidden to speak to her. It was Snow's singular ability to discern a trend at the moment of its inception that

168

established her legend and distinguished her magazine. (Looking at her implacable face at fashion shows, people would whisper, "She *knows*.") *Bazaar* was the first fashion magazine to show both blue jeans and Balenciaga; the first to feature dresses made of cotton (a fabric previously used only for aprons and children's clothes); the first to use action photography (a model in a bathing suit running toward the Hungarian photographer Martin Munkacsi on a beach); the first to use lingerie sketches by an unknown named Christian Dior, whom she knew as "Tian."

Two years into her editorship, Snow turned her art department over to Brodovitch, who had left Russia for Paris in the 1920s and painted stage sets designed by Picasso for Diaghilev's Ballets Russes. As art director of *Bazaar* until 1958, Brodovitch revolutionized the design of magazine layout and graphics, bringing new rhythm and proportion to the pages, interpreting Snow's intrepid vision of fashion and choreographing unpredictable images. A cover might be a slender stilettoed ankle in step with a man's tuxedoed leg, or a woman in summer stripes with her head deemed expendable and cropped out. A tilted column of text in a fashion feature would mimic the slant of the dress it accompanied. There was always, always white space—Diana Vreeland thought Brodovitch's love of white paper must have had its origins in the snow of his native Russia. He believed in the power of photography to communicate with impressionistic techniques—blurred, "bleeding," or stop-action images—along with pen-and-ink illustrations, hand-lettering, and X-rays. At a time when color was unusual in magazines, he used a single second color in contrast with black to great effect. His designs were minimalist during the austere war years, then switched to reflect the hedonism and high spirits of the postwar decade. *Harper's Bazaar* was a laboratory, constantly reexamining and reinventing the magazine medium, using photographers like Hiro and Man Ray and launching the careers of Richard Avedon and Irving Penn, of whom Brodovitch would demand, "Astonish me."

In 1936, according to legend, Snow saw Vreeland dancing in the roof garden of the St. Regis Hotel in white lace Chanel with a rose in her hair and hired her as a fashion editor. Vreeland wrote an outrageously arch column called "Why Don't You . . . ?" in which she made such suggestions as washing a blond child's hair in flat champagne and wearing ballet slippers when leather for shoes was rationed in wartime. She was credited with advising Jacqueline Kennedy to wear a pillbox hat to her husband's inaugural, with coining the phrase "the beautiful people," and with uttering such witticisms as "Pink is the navy blue of India." But she was lured to *Vogue* in 1962, and thereafter *Harper's Bazaar* fell into decline. By 1991, its championship season was long over, but the bitterness of the battle with *Vogue* was still vivid and readily evoked. If *Bazaar* was brought to life again, it would be challenging *Vogue*'s dominance for the first time in thirty years. It could compromise its advertising revenues and undermine its prestige. If *Harper's Bazaar* became a serious contender again, it would mean war between two media giants. Nothing less.

I had just moved with my family yet again, to a new home in Camden Town, an artsy-craftsy area of London, famous for the sprawling weekend street market on the canals and, unfortunately, for IRA bombs going off. We'd knocked down interior walls to make a large open-plan bed and bath suite and outfitted the kitchen with a massive white Aga, the Rolls-Royce of stoves. One evening I was standing under the cellar steps with the washing machine going in the background, when Andrew called me to the phone. It was Jonathan Newhouse, nephew of Condé Nast chairman S. I. Newhouse, calling from Paris, where he ran the European operations of the company.

"I've heard rumors that you're going to New York," he said. "None of it's true," I replied. "We still need to have breakfast," he insisted. "Next Wednesday at Claridge's."

Over poached eggs and coffee that Wednesday, I reiterated that I had no intention of leaving and had not been contacted about any other job. As a sweetener, Jonathan suggested that I was due for a raise and wrote down the amount on a linen napkin. Then he delivered two warnings. "You wouldn't like New York," he said. "There are beggars on every corner, AIDS is rampant, it's a bad place for kids, and if you go to the country, there are ticks and you get Lyme disease." I agreed that New York held no charms for me, and we had a pleasant breakfast, until the waiter refused to let Jonathan sign for the meal on the house account, and he stormed into the cashier's office to have his credit reaffirmed. Then came the clincher. "If you do go," he said, "you will never work for Condé Nast again." I said yes, of course I understood that. Of course I did.

Working for Condé Nast was more than a job. Click-clacking along the blond wood corridors at Vogue House in London, we were a self-satisfied lot. Even the lowliest person on the masthead felt "chosen," and outsiders admitted that just entering the lobby, they felt short of breath, seeing the elite few who somehow knew in their bones how to wear a strand of pearls with a white T-shirt and look fabulous. Once there, many staffers stay for life. The London branch of Condé Nast wasn't part of the rough and dirty world of British journalism, much of it controlled by the press barons Rupert Murdoch and the late Robert Maxwell. Condé Nast was a sealed, self-sufficient microcosm, a culture in which loyalty and discretion were paramount. When I'd entered the Condé Nast hothouse as a humble intern, I was twenty-one. Now I was forty-four and editor of the company's top title in the U.K. So why would I want to leave?

It was time for summer vacation. Andrew and I took the boys for a magical holiday at the Adirondack camp owned by Bruce Weber and his longtime companion, Nan Bush, and finished up staying with Grace Coddington in the Hamptons, just in time for Hurricane Bob. On my last weekend, Grace had a dinner party where Patrick Demarchelier was a guest, and the conversation became a guessing game about the next editor of *Harper's Bazaar.* "England is comfortable and very sweet," he said. "You're doing a nice magazine, but it'll never be better than it is now. If you stay there, you'll just become bourgeois. America is the big time. If you're offered this job, take it."

Patrick had the whole thing planned: I should hire Fabien Baron, the talented French art director who had been at *Interview,* Italian

*Vogue*, and *New York Woman*, but who was then without a magazine. I'd heard about Fabien. I knew he had a scurrilous reputation for provoking battles and getting fired. And I knew I loved his layouts. My mind is full of pictures, not words. I could see Fabien's pages—his bold, colliding, toppling graphics, his profligate use of a whole page for a headline, his letters falling into one another or turned on their side. I began to get a feeling in the pit of my stomach, that excitement of imagining something huge and reckless that can utterly change your life. I'd be severing myself from lifelong colleagues, uprooting my family, fighting Condé Nast. I didn't know how I could do it.

But Patrick said, "If you get Fabien, I'll think about coming with you," and my mind started racing. Even Grace raised an alarmed eyebrow. What Patrick does, simply, is make women look beautiful. His range is unrivaled. There are only a handful of photographers who can determine whether a fashion magazine survives, and I'd need at least one of them to start. I knew that Patrick would bring in the top models and hottest celebrities, that my pages would be filled with arresting images. We'd have material! We'd handpick the world's best fashion editors! We'd forge the most modern, visually arresting magazine in the universe! It would be a crucible of creativity! Together we'd do it!

Well. The next day, when I got back to my comfortable desk in London, the whole idea was just another crazy dinner party conversation with friends when anything seems possible. But I kept getting messages from a man in New York named Frank Farrell, who I thought was a T-shirt salesman: We were having a tedious dispute over a cover photo of five models that some company wanted to emblazon on a T-shirt. So when this nuisance of a man kept phoning and refused to say what he wanted, I figured it was the T-shirt guy and didn't return his calls. Finally he told my secretary he was a friend of Grace Coddington, and I picked up the phone to find out that Frank Farrell was the headhunter hired by Hearst to find an editor for *Bazaar*. He had approached Grace, who said, "You're talking to the wrong person, but I know the right person."

Frank Farrell was a persuasive man, opening the conversation lightly. "Your friend Grace told me you should come to the States," he said. "Would you talk about it over a cup of tea?" The tea was to be taken at the Dorchester Hotel with Frank Bennack, the Hearst CEO, and his deputy Gil Maurer, who were coming to London on business with their British subsidiary, the National Magazine Company. Just to chat, I thought. Perhaps I was being reckless to meet "the enemy" in such a public place, and the inevitable did happen: My production director walked into the bar and looked straight at us. (Either she didn't recognize the opposition or was just discreet, because she never said a word about it.) But there was some defiance in my actions too.

I wasn't thrilled with recent comings and goings at Condé Nast. I was shaken and desperately sad about the early retirement of Richard Hill, the courtly managing director with whom I'd had a long and easy relationship (despite his firm hand on the company purse strings), and I'd started off on the wrong foot with the new editorial director who eventually replaced him. An Old Etonian (i.e., he had attended Britain's most elite school) Nicholas Coleridge was in his early thirties, dapper, relentlessly cheerful, with a clipped, upper-class accent and a confident, somewhat patronizing manner. When he was editor of *Harpers & Queen*, we had a civil enough "How d'you do" relationship, so I thought nothing much of it, in 1989, when he called and asked me to lunch. We chatted inconsequentially. The very next day, his appointment as the new editorial director of Condé Nast U.K. was announced: He was to be my immediate boss. I was incensed—he had failed to say a word about it over lunch. Possibly he'd lost his nerve or had been instructed to keep silent, but either way, it was a rather duplicitous way to behave and not much of a character recommendation, either for Coleridge or for Jonathan Newhouse and the other higher-ups at Condé Nast, whose lapse in courtesy and judgment felt like sabotage. But that wasn't my main problem with Coleridge's appointment. I felt strongly that I didn't need any "help" from someone younger and less experienced than I was. I was thoroughly dismayed by the way his hiring had been presented to me as a fait accompli, and I made my feelings known.

If management thought I'd acquiesce to Coleridge's pre-eminence, they thought wrong. At times like this, the Kelly comes out in me, that family streak of temerity and obstinance in the face of authority. Subtly, I made it clear that he was not welcome on my floor except to attend weekly meetings; I never had to say such a thing to his face. In the foreign service, as I learned from my sister, certain people are known as "mailboxes"—they can be relied upon to carry a message—and that's how I communicated my desires. I don't think they teach the technique at Harvard Business School, but it's a terrific navigational tool for management. I also have my Deep Throats, and I rely dependably on office buzz. That's why I would never have my own private bathroom at work. Too much news gets exchanged in the ladies' room.

There wasn't so much friction as frost between Coleridge and me. One newspaper reported, "It was wonderful to watch how gracefully Liz completely ignored him." The first month his appointment became effective, a note was sent up to my office showing how the masthead should be amended to display Coleridge's title, but gremlins must have gotten into the printing presses, because it just didn't happen, and somehow the oversight made the gossip page in the *Evening Standard*.

But I was beginning to feel I couldn't defend my magazine against all incursions. Again, without my knowledge or consultation, Stephen Quinn, one of Coleridge's former associates from the National Magazine Company, was made British *Vogue*'s publishing director, while Peter Stuart, a reliable, supportive colleague with whom I got on well, was moved to British *GQ*, and Coleridge himself, seemingly the fair-haired boy of Jonathan Newhouse, became managing director of Condé Nast U.K. Other management shuffles added to my growing feeling of isolation and registered as background interference in my daily work. The fun and glory of magazines is being able to hatch ideas, send out talented people to follow them up, and get back something even better than envisioned. I wasn't convinced that the new regime understood and respected British *Vogue* as I did.

I could see that we needed to be aware of the increased competition among fashion magazines and their expanded coverage. What I wouldn't accept was the new management's obsession with the circulation figures of *Marie Claire*, owned by the IPC corporation, launched in 1986. British *Marie Claire* is a magazine that draws in readers with a brew of sex exposés, tight-fitting midpriced clothes, and the diets guaranteed to sculpt those tight places, making for a popular, slightly pornographic fashion magazine that sold quite well. British *Vogue* had never had any real competition, and suddenly in 1991 *Marie Claire* outsold us by 12 percent. But I thought the figures were a false comparison. We had an unassailable upscale position in the market, as unquestionably the most recognized generator of fashion images in the country. I wanted more readers and was doing everything in my power to draw them in, but I was and still am against the inexorable downmarket trend of content and direction that makes magazines end up looking the same. If Condé Nast wanted to compete in the proletarian market, it should launch a new magazine to do that directly, not hijack an already successful one. I was adamant that the way to defend *Vogue*'s territory was to strengthen what we did best. Chasing into the middle ground after *Marie Claire* didn't make any sense to me. Such a strategy came from advertising men thinking about fashion, which is always dangerous.

EVERY NIGHT I'D hash out with Andrew all the pros and cons of moving to New York. The paint was barely dry on our new house, our boys were thriving at school, and my office was peopled with the editors and writers I'd hand-selected, and I loved my fashion friends in London. But neither of us liked the implications of the management changes at Condé Nast. I'd had endless conversations with the new men, but I felt they were set on a course I couldn't support, and my resistance was starting to make my position untenable. If I hadn't had another offer, I surely would have done the expedient thing and tried to meet their demands. But there's a moment when you know you're either part of a team or not. I'd had four happy years as editor of British *Vogue*, and now that I was not so happy, there seemed no reason not to take negotiations with Hearst to the next stage: meeting D. Claeys Bahrenburg, the president of Hearst magazines. The *D* is for Donald, dropped some time ago in favor of the more mysterious and continental-sounding "Claeys." Claeys had joined the company more than ten years before; now he was staking his reputation on pulling *Harper's Bazaar* out of its decline, launching an urgent worldwide search for an editor who could restore its glamour and prestige.

Claeys was in Paris during the time I was covering the pret-a-porter collections in October 1991. Feeling like an inconstant wife, I did some research to find an out-of-the-way lunch spot where we could escape the prying eyes of the usual fashion crowd. I came up with Bofinger, a pretty seafood restaurant with stained glass windows and tiled walls near the Bastille. But I was silly enough to meet Claeys (who is six foot six and hard to hide) at the Hotel Montalambert, where the *Vogue* group was lodged. One of my editors spotted us and asked, "Who's that handsome man you were with?" and I made up something about an old friend of the family.

"Shall we take your car?" I asked after we shook hands.

"I don't have a car," he said, and I went running down the street to retrieve the Condé Nast driver I'd just dismissed, calling even more attention to myself. Claeys's vastly long legs were scrunched up to his chin, even in the back of the Mercedes, on the way to the restaurant. Trying to appear temperate, I ordered Perrier, then said, "I think I need a glass of wine." We both had one and started to relax. As we talked magazines, budgets, readerships, I could see he really understood the editorial product. I was having the kind of conversation I wasn't having at Condé Nast anymore.

Shuttling frantically to and from secret meetings, I was confused, scared, and exhilarated. If I'd been looking for a sign to help me make up my mind, it was right there in the collections, which were saying, rather emphatically, that the 1980s were over. Glitz was giving way to something more sober. Karl Lagerfeld, who had made the Chanel suit a symbol of sex and power by slicing the skirt to thigh-length, suddenly dropped the hem to the knee. It was a shock, a jolt, but I'm always pro-change in fashion. Was I brave enough to apply that attitude to my own life? I knew that British *Vogue* was a good magazine, that I was doing everything I could within the limits of my budget. I also knew that the only place to become a real player in my business was New York. Publishing in Europe is child's play compared to the United States, where the circulation of most magazines is five times that of their European counterparts. In the fashion media, much more advertising is at stake because there are so many more sophisticated readers wanting sophisticated clothes, as well as more retailers and stores where the clothes are sold: Neiman Marcus, Saks Fifth Avenue, Bergdorf Goodman, Bloomingdale's, Macy's, Dayton Hudson, Nordstrom's. And, as my darling husband reminded me, "You're forty-four years old—almost past your 'sell by' date."

I had only two confidants besides Andrew during this period: One was Terry Donovan, whose office right around the corner from Vogue House was where I would go to make clandestine phone calls, the two of us reveling in the secrecy and cowering behind drawn blinds like Maxwell Smart and Agent 99. My other ally was Grace Coddington, happily ensconced at American *Vogue*, whose advice was "Get your ass over here." She had no qualms about the two of us being friendly competitors. Such arrangements are more common than you'd think. But I needed something concrete against which to calculate the risk.

In early November, I went to the New York collections as usual and met Frank Farrell face to face for the first time, along with his partner Jane Phinn, for breakfast at the Carlyle Hotel. "You know," he said, "you'll have to make up your mind." I confessed that I was completely confused. "What you must do is write it all down," he said, "everything you want to do and everything you need to do it. Then you'll know, and Hearst will know too." So in between shows, in my hotel suite, I set it down in an eighteen-page document. I wanted assurance that I would be editing the magazine by myself, without interference. I wanted a serious budget to cover the cost of sending fashion teams to the collections several times a year. I wanted world-class photographers and writers. I wanted guarantees about a promotional budget for the relaunch. I wanted the actual dimensions of the magazine changed to the newer, slightly smaller size that felt more modern and fit better into women's purses and supermarket pockets. And I wanted to abolish the perennial "Over 40 and Fabulous" stories. As I wrote down my requests, I could feel the excitement of momentous opportunity—a professional clean slate and a whole new life for my family. But I still needed a push, in one direction or the other. And so I made an appointment to see my ultimate boss, S. I. Newhouse himself.

Si is unlike any mogul I have ever known. Small and quiet, rarely displaying any emotion beyond a Mona Lisa half-smile, he is a man camouflaged by his low-profile demeanor: You could pass him in a corridor without ever registering his presence, let alone knowing that this is one of the wealthiest men on the planet. He makes few social appearances and arrives for work at five A.M., traits that only serve to make him more enigmatic and daunting. Our contact had been sporadic but cordial. When he visited London, he never made an appointment. If I knew he was in town, I just stayed by my desk in case he showed up. Sometimes he did, sometimes he didn't. When he did, we'd have a brief chat about business. He never said much. Once he wrote me a note saying he'd liked an issue.

That Tuesday I took the elevator up to Si's office at Condé Nast headquarters on Madison Avenue. He was sitting in a plain white room, behind a plain black desk, with magazines strewn all over the floor. I took a deep breath and started talking. I tried to explain my unhappiness resulting from the departure of so many of the people I'd worked with for years in London. All he said was "I see" and "Right," never indicating whether he liked British *Vogue* or the job I was doing with it. If I hadn't had another job offer in the background, I would have left his office feeling thoroughly dejected. As it was, I was pricked by sadness and anger at being so apparently unheard. If he had just dropped his habitual inscrutability for one moment to give me and British *Vogue* a vote of confidence,

I would have happily stayed on. But by the time I walked out on the street, I knew exactly what I was going to do.

"Take me to Nine Fifty-nine Eighth Avenue," I said to the driver of my hired car.

New York drivers know everything. "That's the Hearst building," he said.

I'd arranged a meeting with Claeys Bahrenburg that I could have canceled if I had had a more constructive encounter with Si Newhouse. Instead, I was submitting that eighteen-page document detailing everything I saw as necessary to bringing *Bazaar* around. I knew from watching Anna Wintour take over at British *Vogue* how difficult it was to inherit a recalcitrant, embittered staff. The most important item on my list was really an ultimatum, one that sounded ruthless but contained the seeds of success for revamping a magazine.

"Do you realize that you'll have to let a lot of people go?" I asked. "The magazine is stodgy, complacent, uninspired. I need carte blanche to choose people with vision and drive. It'll be tough. You'll have to ignore what anyone says, inside the company or in the press. But I need that guarantee."

"Okay," said Claeys. "I don't see a problem there."

This *was* the big time, and when I returned to London, Andrew and I decided there was a lot at stake in this move, so after consulting with Terry Donovan we hired an international lawyer to hammer out my contract. But I trusted Andrew's instincts, his antennae, and it was important that he join me when I flew back to New York a few weeks later to meet with Claeys. Grace had warned me, "You're bound to run into somebody who will put two and two together and know why you're there. You've got to think of an alibi." We decided to say that it was an anniversary trip (never mind that we were married in July), combined with Christmas shopping. We walked into the British Airways terminal at Heathrow Airport and heard "Liz! What are you doing here?" It was Marina Schiano, then fashion editor of *Vanity Fair*, exactly the sort of person who was wired in to all the gossip. We fed her the alibi, and she seemed to bite. In New York, Andrew and Claeys bonded over drinks while I did some actual shopping. I was in the Ralph

Lauren store on Madison Avenue when I heard a voice saying "Liz . . ." It was Helen O'Hagan, then the public relations director of Saks Fifth Avenue.

"What are you doing in New York?" she asked.

"Shopping," I said innocently.

"Yeah, right," she snorted. Helen was good friends with Ellin Saltzman, then the fashion director of Bergdorf Goodman; I knew that Helen would tell Ellin, and it would be only a short time before the secret was out. Billy Norwich, who wrote the gossip column "Page Six" for the *New York Post* at the time, was the first to call and ask me to confirm that I would be the editor-in-chief of *Harper's Bazaar*. I persuaded him to withhold the story, promising him the first interview when we went public.

Back in London in mid-December, I was working on my résumé. I'd never had a proper résumé before. No one would have been the least bit interested in the chronicles of Elizabeth Tilberis before this, and it would have consisted of one word: *Vogue*, where I'd been all my professional life. But I still hadn't signed the contract. Claeys was calling me constantly, from his house, his car, even from a cell phone on the deck of his boat, moored for the winter outside his house at Orient Point, Long Island. At Christmastime, I gave a party for the British *Vogue* staff at our new house, and as I was going to the door to greet Terry Donovan and his wife, a messenger on a motorbike drove up with a large envelope. Terry signed for it and came up the stairs grinning.

"Do I know what this is?" he asked.

"Yes, you do," I answered. He was thrilled to be the bearer of my contract.

Over the New Year's holiday, we rented a house in Somerset to be near my parents, and one day Nick Coleridge called me there. The gossip columnist of "Londoner's Diary" in the *Evening Standard* had called him to verify the rumor that I was going to Hearst.

"It's absolutely untrue, Nick," I said. "I'd let you know." It's awful to prevaricate like that, but I still hadn't signed. I told another lie too: Because I was afraid that I might be prevented from

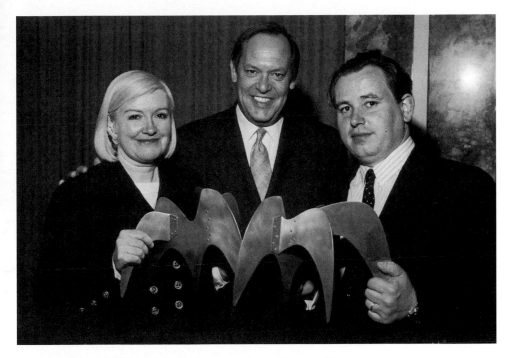

Winning the ASME award: me, then president of Hearst Magazine Division Claeys Bahrenburg, and Fabien Baron. April 1993. *(Photo by Larry Lettera.)*

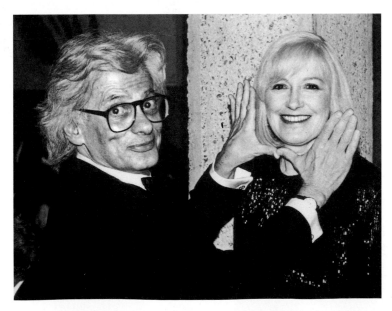

Being "framed" by master photographer Richard Avedon, at the Whitney exhibition opening of *Richard Avedon Evidence, 1944–1994*, which *Bazaar* hosted. March 1994, after my diagnosis with ovarian cancer. *(Photo by Arthur Elgort.)*

Andrew and me
with Sam and
Sophie on the
beach in the
Hamptons with my
own short hair.

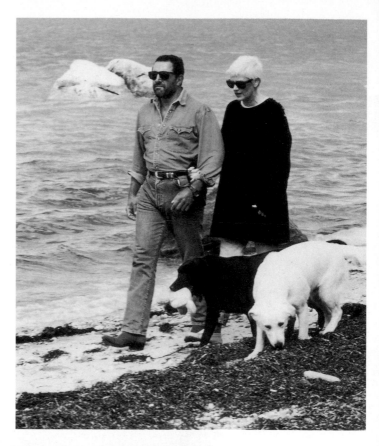

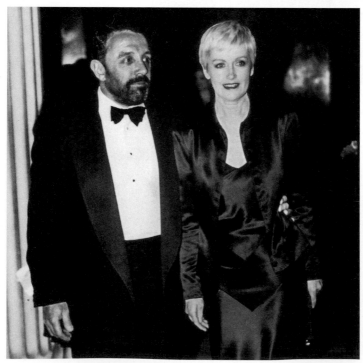

Andrew and me,
starting to go out
again on the social
circuit after my
chemo treatments.

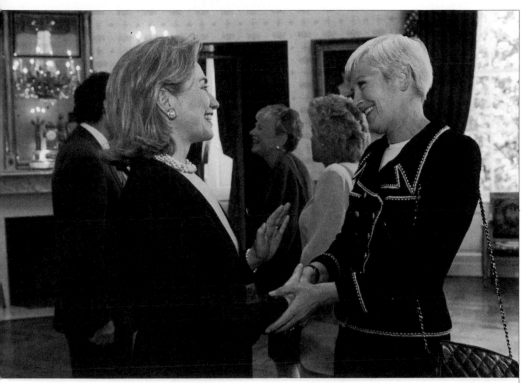

To Liz Tilberis
With best wishes, and appreciation —
Hillary Rodham Clinton

At the White House with the first lady,
Hillary Rodham Clinton, in 1994. She
hosted a cocktail party for The Pediatric
AIDS Foundation, a kickoff for the Kids 4
Kids event in New York City later that year.

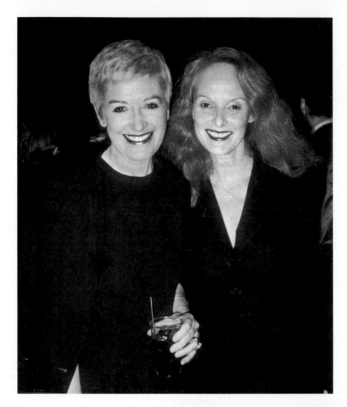

Grace and me at the Calvin Klein after-runway party in November 1994.

*Opposite:* Backshot of H.R.H. The Princess of Wales and me leaving the stage where she presented me with the 1994 CFDA Special Award in January 1995.

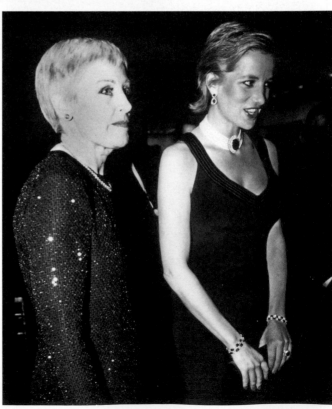

H.R.H. The Princess of Wales and me at the CFDA reception.

To a roy special lady . . . . .

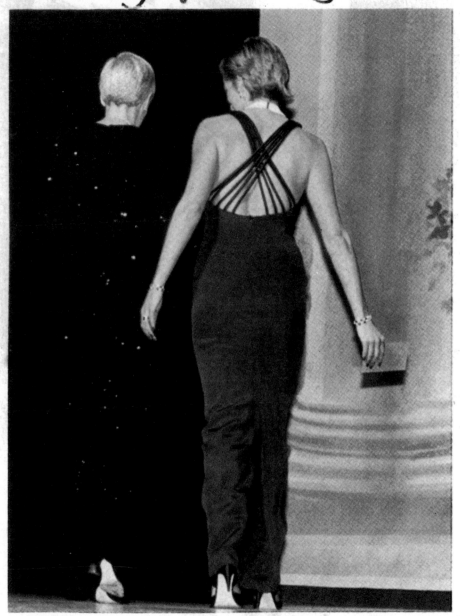

with fondest love from Diana *.
1995.

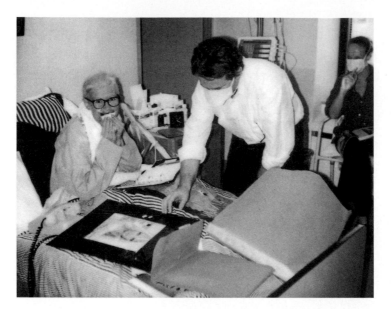

At the hospital, during my bone marrow treatment in August 1995, with art director Paul Eustace, choosing that wishy-washy cover logo—Grace is sitting on the window sill.

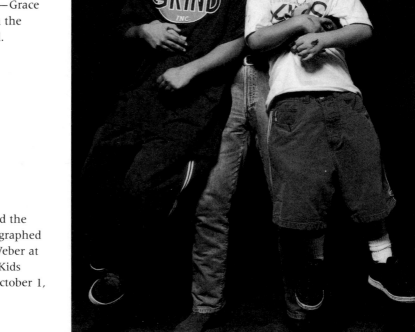

Andrew and the boys photographed by Bruce Weber at the Kids 4 Kids event on October 1, 1995.

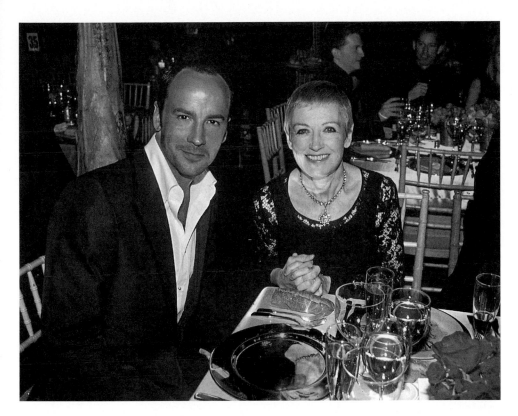

With Tom Ford in
my Gucci outfit at
the CFDA awards,
February 1996.
*(Photo by Patrick
McMullan.)*

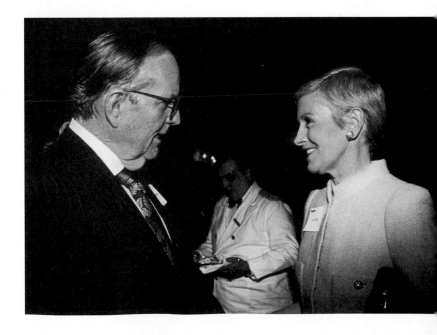

Wearing a Chanel
couture jacket,
talking with Mr.
Randolph Hearst.
*(Photo by Blaivas.)*

How are you?
(well I hope)
Where are you?
With all my love Karl

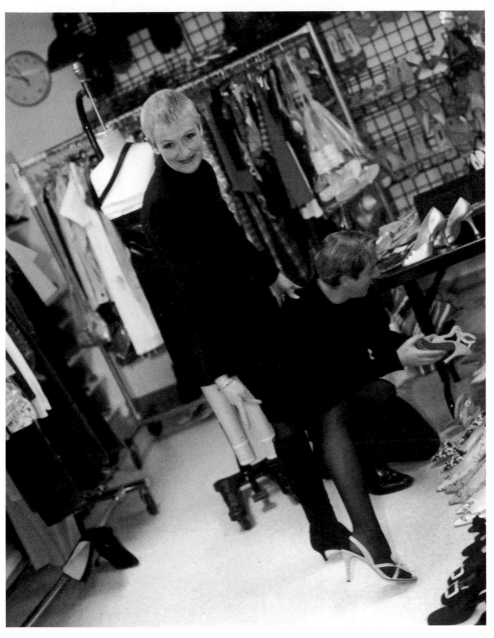

In the fashion closet at the magazine, my favorite place, trying on shoes.
*(Photo by Michel Arnaud.)*

*Opposite:* Karl Lagerfeld's drawing from August 1996, my head turned into a question mark, while he wonders "How are you? Where are you?"

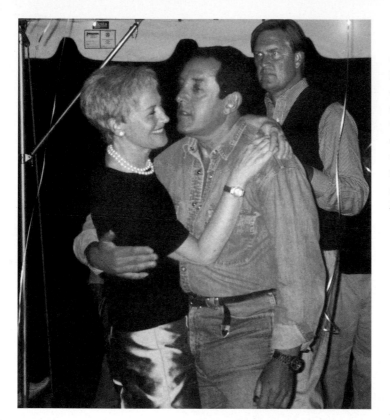

At our twenty-fifth
wedding anniversary
party: having a dance
with Andrew to Dr.
John's band, despite
my wig all askew.

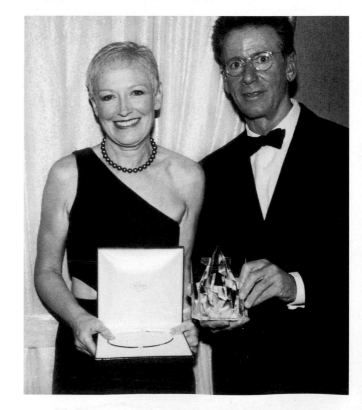

At the Fashion Group
International's Night
of Stars, where I was
presented with an
award by Calvin Klein.
September 16, 1996.
Here, with Calvin Klein.

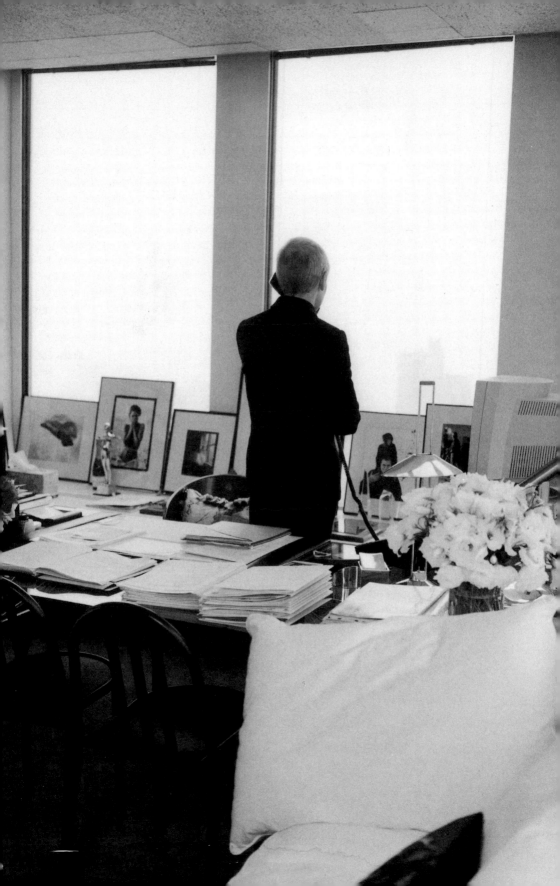

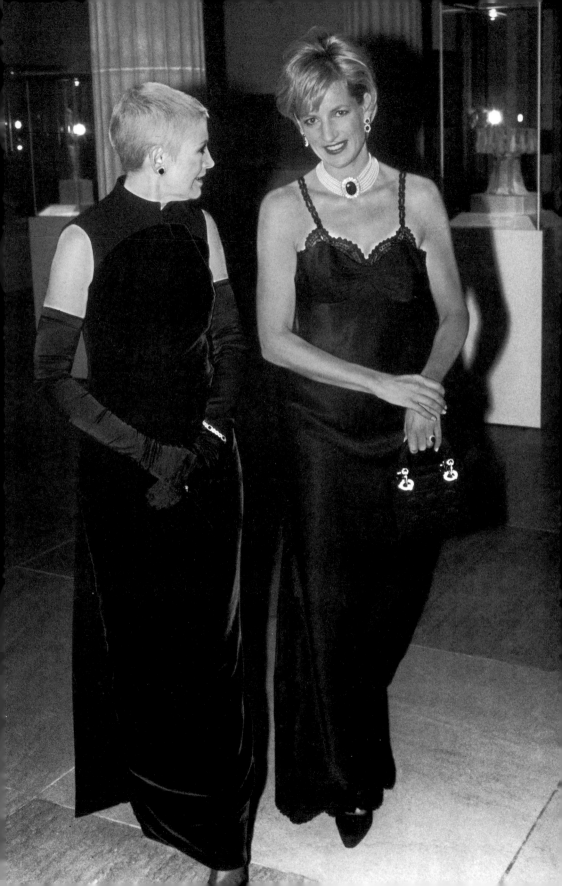

*Opposite:* Diana, Princess of Wales, and me walking to dinner at the Metropolitan Museum of Art's Costume Institute. December 9, 1996. *(Photo by Don Pollard.)*

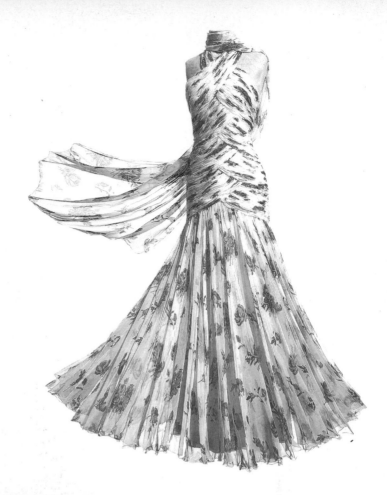

The Catherine Walker gown that the Princess of Wales auctioned at Christie's and *Harper's Bazaar* purchased on June 25, 1997. We donated it to the Metropolitan Museum of Art's Costume Institute. The gown was worn by the princess on an official visit to Nigeria in 1988. *(Photo by Dennis Golonka.)*

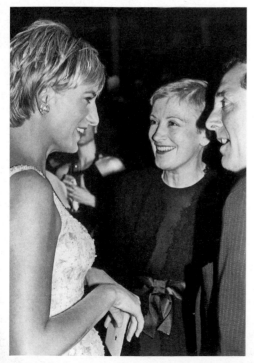

At the Christie's reception to benefit AIDS Crisis Trust two evenings before the auction of the Princess of Wales's dresses. Andrew and I greet Diana, Princess of Wales. It was the last time I would ever see her. June 23, 1997. *(Photo by Daisey Donovan.)*

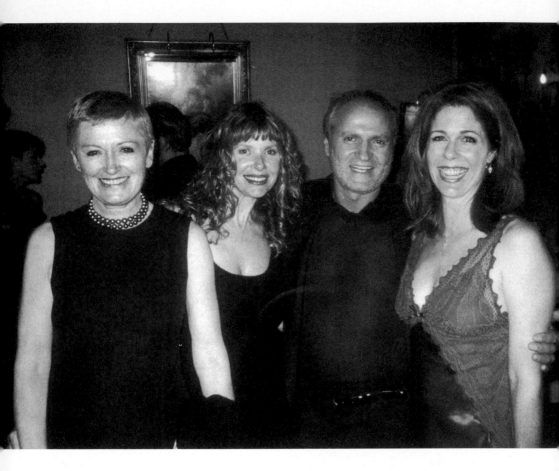

July 6, 1997, at the Versace Couture show with actress Kate Capshaw; the late, and dearly missed, Gianni Versace; and actress Rita Wilson in Paris. It was the last time I would see Gianni.

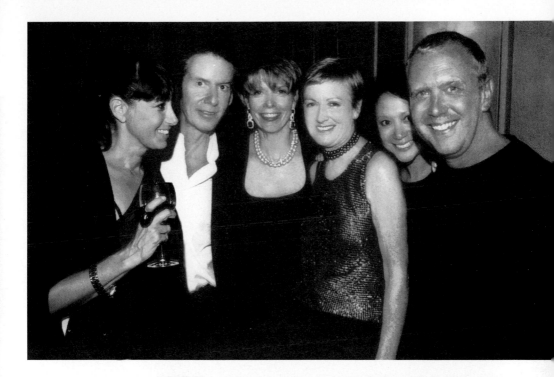

At my fiftieth birthday party thrown by Cathie Black, president of Hearst Magazines Division, at Gertrude's the day I returned from the funeral of Diana, Princess of Wales. With, from left: Donna Karan, Calvin Klein, Cathie Black, Jeannette Chang, and Michael Kors. *(Photo by Doug Goodman.)*

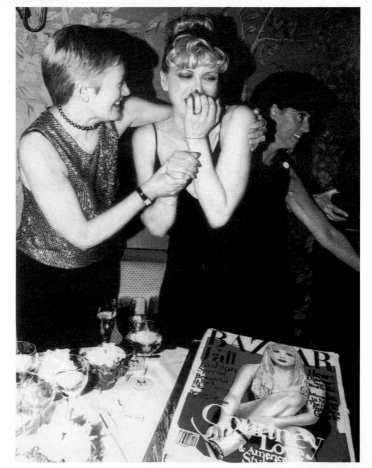

With Courtney Love, our September 1997 cover girl. *(Photo by Doug Goodman.)*

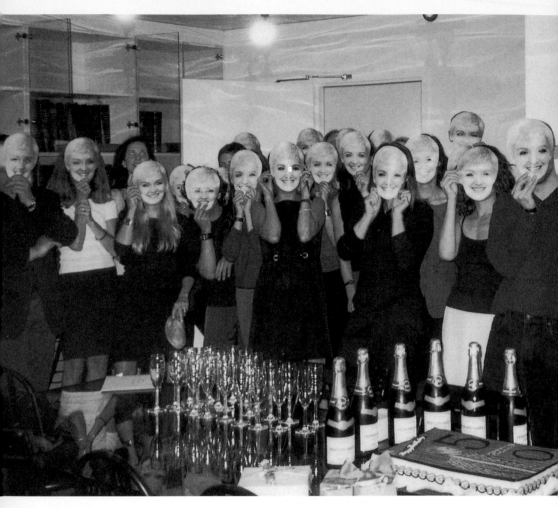

My surprise fiftieth birthday party that my
staff threw for me. The entire staff wore
"Liz" masks as I walked into the room.
*(Photo by Dennis Golonka.)*

removing my things—my Rolodex, files, bound volumes of British *Vogue*—once I announced my departure, I said that I was going to have the office painted and started sending boxes home "for safekeeping." Sitting in my lawyer's office a few days later, finally putting my signature on all those carbon copies, was almost anti-climactic, as six months of negotiations were dispensed with in a few moments. But driving in to work immediately after New Year on the morning I was going to resign felt like graduation—with the feeling of melancholy at leaving the comfort and familiarity of my home for more than twenty years, together with the thrill of contemplating the next stage. But most keenly I felt the betrayal of my team in the wake of my good fortune: Another editor would come in, and some of them would get fired. That's the way things go. Heads roll. For the heads that were to roll on my account, I felt terrible. For myself, I felt terrified. I knew I was taking on a Herculean task.

When I got to the office, I called Nick Coleridge. "Can you spare me a couple of minutes?" I asked.

"Certainly," he said and came upstairs. I closed the doors, and we sat at my table.

"Nick," I said, "I'm resigning."

"Is it because of me?" he asked.

"I've been offered the job at *Harper's Bazaar*," I said.

He smiled, said "Oh," then a few words of polite congratulations before he went off to tell management, and I wrote resignation memos. I was spared Jonathan Newhouse's lectures and never heard from Si Newhouse. I called the senior editors in to my office one by one, then groups from each department. Most were quiet, happy for me but scared for themselves. Some had lived through the last sea change and knew that very few manage to cling to the sides of the ship. In the middle of this weepy day, the man who'd been hired to landscape the garden at our new home arrived for an appointment I'd forgotten to cancel, bearing sheets of paper proposing azalea bushes and tea roses. "So sorry," I had to tell him, "we're leaving the country."

The next few weeks were a blur. I needed the kind of visa that allowed me to work in the United States and bring my husband and children. Andrew was supervising the hasty packing of our household and would join me later. The children were a little apprehensive, at ages ten and six trying to appraise the loss of friends, schools, and their beloved soccer. (Chris was still too young to appreciate the change, and Robbie was bribed with the promise of a puppy in New York.) At my going-away party in Covent Garden, hosted by *Vogue* and the British Fashion Council, the monumental cake was a Liz Tilberis figure as the Statue of Liberty dressed in a red Chanel suit, standing atop a stack of books with titles such as *It's a Learning Curve* by Andrew Tilberis, and *I Did It Her Way* by the Princess of Wales. The princess came for my last official appearance, as cochair of a charity premiere: *The Prince of Tides* meets the Princess of Wales. I was filled with pride when Robbie presented the princess with flowers and Chris gave her a program. Diana sat next to the film's star and director, Barbra Streisand, and there was some discreet tittering between them during the love scenes with Nick Nolte, who was sitting next to me, sound asleep. The next day I was departing England for good, and my whole family came for a grand send-off—my parents, my closest friends, their children, my godchildren. But the hardest part of all was saying goodbye to my father, his mind too frail to even register that I'd be gone.

# 12

ON JANUARY 6, 1992, I was named editor-in-chief of *Harper's Bazaar*. Media-watchers rubbed their collective hands with glee and said, "Let the games begin." News of my appointment was announced the next day in the *New York Times* under the headline "Brits in High Places." Several top publishing jobs in America had recently been Anglicized, not just with the half-English, half-American Anna Wintour at *Vogue*, but also Tina Brown (then editor of *Vanity Fair* and later *The New Yorker*), her husband, Harold Evans (founding editor of *Condé Nast Traveler*, later publisher of Random House, and now editorial director and vice-chairman of the *Daily News* and the *Atlantic Monthly*), and James Truman (editor of *Details* and subsequently editorial director of Condé Nast). It was a point, a sore point, that was to be hammered home over the next year. (*Spy* magazine put it so archly: "The new British invasion: How American publishing has been taken over by people with charming accents and bad teeth.")

The *Times* also hinted at the other angle that would keep the press endlessly entertained for months to come: my relationship with Anna Wintour. I didn't get any flowers of congratulations from her, but she made a gracious response to the press queries: "The more British editors, the better," she declared. No matter what either of us said to play down our personal rivalry, the press on both sides of the Atlantic was intent on setting up a catfight. Anna versus Liz, *Vogue* versus *Bazaar*, Condé Nast versus Hearst— it was far too juicy to resist.

The headlines began even before I left England. "Liz and Anna Wage Savage Frock War," screamed the London *Daily Express*. "Fashion Queens Fall Out," announced the *Daily Mail*. "Clash of the Titans," boomed the *Los Angeles Times*. And in *New York* magazine: "The duel between Tilberis and Wintour is being taken as seriously as other great dustups in recent corporate culture, like Herb Siegel of Chris-Craft versus Steve Ross of Warner, or record moguls David Geffen and Walter Yetnikoff." Over the next few months, the speculation got so outrageous that Billy Norwich wrote in the *New York Post*, "In a male-dominated press, women are pitted against each other like Alexis and Krystle on 'Dynasty.' It's a real turn-on for the men to see women fighting."

All I knew was that I wanted to make *Harper's Bazaar* the most beautiful fashion magazine in the world. It was as simple, and as huge, and as daunting as that. The plan was that Tony Mazzola would retire with the June 1992 issue. I'd caretake July and August, then debut with September, the blockbuster issue that announces the fall collections and attracts the heftiest number of advertising pages. That gave me little time to select my dream team and create the most elegant fashion magazine I could conceive of.

I'd done my research via the fashion grapevine and learned that there were good people at *Bazaar* I wanted to keep, and five years later, some of them are still with me as my senior staff. But the unpleasant fact of life was that many of the staff had to go, in the same sort of housecleaning that takes place whenever a new executive is installed in any enterprise, whether it's magazines or banking. Years before, Mazzola himself had fired a young editor named Anna Wintour from *Harper's Bazaar*.

Claeys Bahrenburg asked me to drop in at the office one day to say hello and reassure the staff that everything was going to be okay, when I knew perfectly well that everything was *not* going to be okay. I reluctantly complied, and, sure enough, we proceeded to fire several top staff at the magazine. The changes were dramatized in an industry newsletter as a "bloodbath," and some of the people over forty threatened an age discrimination suit—never mind that I was nearly forty-five myself. Awful as I felt, being responsible for people losing their jobs, I stuck to my guns over the importance of bringing in a whole new creative team.

Since I had not yet received my U.S. visa, I could not officially move to New York, so I effectively had to be in two places at once. The only way I could approximate that feat was to take the Concorde back and forth each week, a schedule that let me put two extra hours in the day, leaving London at eleven a.m. and arriving in New York at nine a.m. I moved into the Carlyle Hotel and led a schizophrenic life, living out of a suitcase but expected to look smart, waking up and literally not knowing where I was, figuring out the few moments in the day when Andrew, Robbie, Chris, and I would all be awake and able to visit by phone. Mazzola would remain in place for several months, so there was no question of my moving into the *Bazaar* offices right away, and I was given borrowed space at *Esquire*. At that point, the new *Harper's Bazaar* consisted of me and my assistant, Anna Cryer, who had left British *Vogue* on the promise of a job in New York, working from the dining room table at our house in Camden Town until we moved.

Almost immediately my fax machine was tied up with missives from Richard Avedon, the living legend who was the prototype for the Fred Astaire character in *Funny Face* and had begun his career at *Bazaar* in the 1940s. We went to breakfast at Rumpelmayer's on Central Park, and Avedon's ideas for change came out in a torrent, the scope of his vision reaching so far beyond the realm of photography that it was obvious the role befitting his talent and seniority would be creative director. Bowled over by that idea as I was, I didn't think Avedon would want to be a team player, and I didn't know how the two of us would work together, where I would fit into his all-encompassing view of the new *Bazaar*. One morning I called Claeys Bahrenburg, feeling as if I wanted to hand somebody else the reins of my life and say, "Here, you drive for a while." My voice was weak with anxiety.

"It's amazing that Avedon would want to work with us," I squeaked, "but I'm not sure it's right."

"It's your call," replied Claeys. "But if he's creative director, I'm not sure you'll be able to edit." I knew that, but I needed to hear it articulated. Passing up the chance to work with Avedon was a frightening choice to make, like a rookie saying "No thanks" to batting practice with Babe Ruth.

I also eliminated Grace Coddington from the running. Ever since I'd taken the job, Grace and I had talked about the possibility of working together again, but the dynamic of our relationship in the past had been that she was my boss, and I didn't think she'd want to reverse those roles. We decided that you can never really go back and that it wouldn't matter if I was at *Bazaar* and she was at *Vogue*. She was happy there, and we trusted our ancient friendship enough to figure out a comfortable compromise between our usual wont to dish and a more sensible policy of "Don't ask, don't tell." My dream team of photographers was a short list: Patrick Demarchelier, with his journalistic talent in documenting fashion; Peter Lindbergh, whose work had such wistful romance; and Steven Meisel, who took extravagantly glamorous pictures. If I got any one of these key players, I knew that the pages would be filled with gorgeous images, the buzz would be so strong that models and celebrities would line up to get in, and we'd be hot as hell. A small hitch: All three were *Vogue* people. Condé Nast did not give contracts to photographers at the time, but Si Newhouse made it plain that his company was not into sharing and let it be known, via the jungle drums, that photographers who worked for *Bazaar* would be banned by every Condé Nast publication worldwide, a threat that had the effect of upping the financial ante instantaneously. People who chose to work for me were making this big career commitment because they were in love with the project, with being part of a team creating, from scratch, a magazine that would look and operate differently from *Vogue*.

186

My husband and sons, still packing up our lives in London, were coming over for a two-week visit in February, and the Carlyle was far too expensive for such a clan. Eleanor Lambert, the grande dame of fashion public relations who created the International Best-Dressed List, offered us the presidential suite at the St. Regis Hotel, another of her clients. It looked like Xanadu: a massive marble foyer leading to an even more massive living room, a dining room fit for a state banquet, and a suite of bedrooms. The boys could practically rollerblade in the bathtub and each gained several pounds from mini-bar macadamia nuts and room-service sundaes. Andrew joined me in my first public appearance as the newly named editor of *Bazaar* at the awards ceremony for the Council of Fashion Designers of America at Lincoln Center. It was freezing cold that night, but I shunned a coat to make an entrance in a short black Chanel suit, with Andrew on one side and Claeys Bahrenburg on the other, escorting Lauren Hutton. The paparazzi went crazy, and I felt like the Three Faces of Eve: generous congratulations and good-luck wishes from the designers, worrisome glances from the *Bazaar* staff, and glowers from Condé Nast people.

I was getting used to the cold shoulder: In the midst of my negotiations for my new team came the January Paris couture, and with no staff yet in place, I found myself sitting all alone in the front row at the shows, highly exposed and conspicuous. The existing *Bazaar* staff was there, pointing and whispering, and Condé Nast-ers publicly snubbed me as well, perhaps spooked by the potential consequences of being seen talking to an adversary. Meanwhile half the fashion editors in the world were calling my hotel room and pressing notes into my hands, pleading for jobs. One woman followed me into a bathroom and stuck her résumé under the door of the stall.

Patrick Demarchelier had been teasing Fabien Baron, calling him weekly to say, "Have I got a job for you!" and then refusing to tell him where. Fabien and his wife, Sciascia Gambaccini, whom he'd met at Italian *Vogue*, had set up Baron & Baron, a design and advertising agency, but when Patrick finally confessed where the great job would be, Fabien's first reaction was, "Ah! How cool!

187

Bringing back *Bazaar*!" We met for lunch in January at a midtown Italian restaurant called Bice, and after the antipasto, it was a foregone conclusion that I'd hire him as creative director. Alexey Brodovitch had been the biggest influence of Fabien's life, and my ideal was to run the art department as Brodovitch had, as a workshop for creative talent. We left the restaurant light-headed with possibilities, and Fabien accepted the job on the condition that he could keep Baron & Baron going, which he did. When I met his wife, I was so impressed with her portfolio of work and feisty personality that I hired her too, as a fashion editor. We had a tiny team with which to start.

Paul Cavaco was a left-field contender—not an editor at all but a public relations agent. His company, Keeble, Cavaco and Duka, had handled the staging of fashion shows for clients such as Gianni Versace and the styling of advertising campaigns for Barneys. Both of his business partners had recently died: his ex-wife, Kezia Keeble, of breast cancer, and her second husband, John Duka, of AIDS. Paul was ready for a change and a new challenge. At the time, he was styling Madonna's soon-to-be-notorious book, *Sex*, photographed by Steven Meisel. When he called and asked to come talk with me at the St. Regis, he pointed to a large scratch in the dining room table. "Madonna did that in her stilettos," he said dryly. Possessed of an encyclopedic knowledge of images from *Bazaar*'s greatest years, Paul was dying to "be" Diana Vreeland, even selling his stake in his own company to join us as a fashion director.

The idea of *two* fashion directors was unusual, but we needed a powerful team to turn *Bazaar* around, and I had another admirable candidate. There was a new regime at Calvin Klein, and Tonne Goodman, who'd been vice-president of advertising there, decided to leave the company. Tonne's work on campaigns such as Eternity perfume had the kind of simple, pristine, and utterly modern look I wanted to achieve in *Bazaar*, and the timing was perfect. I never really interviewed her, or Paul either. In filling such positions, it's all about reputation. These people come with their medals pinned to their chest, even if the previous job description was somewhat different. You cannot interview a fashion director. You don't have a conversation about clothes, and you don't say, "This is the way *Bazaar* is going to be." You know what they've done before you ever meet, and if you're not allergic to each other at that meeting, you hire them and just let them work.

Then we had to start talking money with the photographers, and every time we made an offer, *Vogue* made a counteroffer. It was a poker game, played at a corporate level, our ace in the hole being "creative freedom," the one perquisite those guys craved most. Anna Wintour's style, as I knew from working with her, is prescriptive: She tells people what she wants, and they have to come back with it. If it's not what she had in mind, she kills it. That's one way of editing, but not mine. I kept repeating that *Bazaar* was going to be far more democratic, a think tank. No pictures of girls with tulips running in the street. But I realized that hiring photographers for *Bazaar* was going to cost Hearst a couple of million dollars. It was an unprecedented situation, but we were changing history. Even cool-hand Claeys was beginning to sweat, sprinting down the hallway clutching my memos and yelling, "We can't afford this!" Finally he and I went to see Frank Bennack, the man holding the purse strings of the Hearst Corporation, and outlined my expensive plans, asking whether the company would keep its nerve. "Liz," he said, "I'm proud to be part of the great debacle." That gave me the courage I needed to keep wooing the photographers.

Peter Lindbergh is a handsome, debonair German—women were always falling in love with him—and we had a long, easy rapport: Our past adventures included driving through Deauville with Stephanie Seymour, risking arrest by playing T-Rex at top decibel, and freezing on Miami Beach, with Cindy Crawford so cold that Peter stripped down to his underpants so he would have the same goosebumps. He finally agreed that the prospect of reinventing *Bazaar* was too good to pass up. When his agent called and said, "He's ready to sign," I arranged to fly to Paris for one night with his contract in hand, arriving at JFK to discover Si Newhouse waiting to board the same flight. "My wife would love to meet you," he said affably, and we exchanged pleasantries, both of us knowing that he was going to Paris in the hope of quashing the deal. But I knew that I'd won that round before we ever left New York. Peter's contract was signed with champagne and kisses at a café on the Boulevard St.-Germain.

Meisel kept us hanging on. It was hard to know which way he would go. At one point, he seemed so close to joining that I invited him to a meeting in my dreary temporary office with my tiny team to talk magazine strategy. It was a dramatic day in the city. Los Angeles had erupted after the Rodney King trial, and there was concern about copycat rioting in New York, so most places of business shut down early. The streets were eerily deserted, except for a heavy police presence—when we went to Cipriani's in the Sherry Netherland Hotel for lunch, we could have waltzed down Fifth Avenue. But it became clear that Meisel wasn't as decided as I thought when his lunch "date" showed up: the flamboyant, heavily bejeweled *Vogue* fashion editor Carlyne Cerf de Dudzeele, who'd been included in earlier talks about coming to *Bazaar*, which had not panned out. When I saw her, I knew Meisel was keeping his ties to *Vogue*. He'd done much of his best work for Italian *Vogue* with Fabien Baron as art director, but it turned out that Franca Sozzani, the editor-in-chief, felt she'd "discovered" him and caused a major scene over the possibility of losing him.

"Look," Fabien told him persuasively, "there's a train leaving this station. There won't be another opportunity like this for ten years, if ever in our lifetime. Any number of fashion magazines might start up, but what are they compared to *Harper's Bazaar*? Think about the name. Think about the provenance. Think about the fun. It's not going to happen again." But Meisel decided he couldn't give up Italian *Vogue*.

Fabien was right: It *would* have been fun, but what counted more than anything was that I get Patrick Demarchelier, the man at the top of my list. I could see exactly how painful the decision was for him: leaving the company where he had earned his living since he was a kid. But I knew he was feeling limited by the repetitive work he was being given at *Vogue*. One Saturday morning, I went to his Manhattan apartment just after he'd

190

returned from a job in Paris; he was lying on the sofa in a bathrobe.

"We can't do anything today," he said with great weariness, "because I left the contract in Paris."

"Not to worry," I said, quick as a flash. "I've got a copy in my bag." Patrick knew the moment had arrived, but he was so nervous he had to sign from a prone position. With that swipe of the pen, the team was in place: the new kids on the block, the underdogs, the ones who were going to shake things up. I left Patrick's apartment walking on air, and drove straight to JFK to greet my family on their permanent arrival in New York.

All the action taking place in early 1992 was rocket fuel for gossip. By the time I went to Milan in March for the fall collections, I had company. When Fabien sat down in the empty seat next to me at the Armani show, there was a collective intake of breath, a split second of silence, and then an almighty outbreak of yakkety-yakking. We'd broken cover. The publicity peaked in April on the cover of *New York* magazine: a photograph of Anna Wintour and me with the blaring headline, "War of the Poses—*Bazaar*'s New Liz Takes On *Vogue*'s Anna," our faces outlined as if we were the cover girls on our own magazines. The photograph had been taken at *Vogue*'s hundredth-anniversary party at the New York Public Library in March. It was civilized of Condé Nast to invite me, a *Vogue* lifer until a couple of months before, although the air was fraught with tension as I approached the receiving line to shake hands with my former employers. Half of me was terrified, but the other half likes a challenge. I congratulated Si Newhouse on the choice of my replacement at British *Vogue*: Alexandra Shulman, whom I'd hired as a features editor and who since had become the editor of British GQ. Anna and I embraced politely and smiled for the photographers, both of us knowing that such a picture was strategically important. She had to be perceived as above the fray, unthreatened by the competition. From my point of view, the more people knew about *Harper's Bazaar*, the better.

By April of 1992, my husband and sons had joined me in New York, but the pet portion of the family was detained. Our first cat had appeared on our doorstep shortly before we adopted Robbie, as a dark blob that I thought was a pile to avoid stepping in, until I realized that the pile had eyes. She died when the boys were little, and we buried her in the backyard. As we were conducting the appropriate memorial service, another kitten appeared on the stone wall behind our garden, rather like a designated mourner representing the animal kingdom at this otherwise all-human funeral. And he never left. We sent word around the neighborhood that a stray had been found, but nobody ever claimed him. We called him Gazza, the nickname for a soccer player named Paul Gascoyne on the British team in the World Cup that year. We lost a cat, we gained a cat—a bit spooky but a rather tidy sequence. When Andrew was doing the final packing for New York, Gazza disappeared, probably in protest, and was rescued by our nanny. He lived with a friend until I retrieved him on my next trip to London and brought him back to New York on the Concorde, which was not to his liking, and everybody at Kennedy Airport knew about it. I could hear his howls long before I saw him. He was even less pleased to greet our two new labradors, Samantha and Sophie. (When we had gone to the breeder in Wainscott, Long Island, for Robbie's promised puppy, Christopher had started crying that he wanted one too.)

We quickly discovered the favorite spot in Manhattan of expatriate Britons homesick for the peculiar foods of the motherland, a shop downtown called Myers of Keswick. There we found meat pies, sausages, and Scotch eggs; the vegetable extract called Marmite that we put on bread (an American friend says it smells like the bottom of an aquarium); an effervescent orange drink called Lucozade; Heinz baked beans (which are *not* the same as the American variety); Bisto gravy browning, and Jaffa Cakes: cookies that have chocolate on top, sponge on the bottom, and jam inside. I had to reinvent many things my children liked that were impossible to duplicate with local ingredients. They soon discovered American delicacies and we relied less on Myers, but supermarket shopping was a magical mystery tour for me: The brand names and packaging are completely different, from dishwashing powder to butter, and what Americans call English breakfast tea is not what English people drink for breakfast. I'm still scared of butchers, after I ordered a leg of lamb and received meat that was "butterflied" and denuded of all its fat. I wouldn't know what to do with something butterflied, and the gorgeous fat is what turns brown and becomes gravy (with the help of Bisto). Periodically I caused titters at the butcher when I called and asked for a joint rather than a roast.

We had moved to temporary quarters at an apartment-hotel called the Bristol Plaza. The boys liked the rooftop pool, but we were getting discouraged about ever finding a permanent residence. We were used to the size and style of a family house in Britain, while many New Yorkers live in what much of the world would consider closet space. Fabien Baron had found his apartment through a realtor named Linda Stein who used to work in the music business and had a reputation for shepherding "difficult" clients such as Sylvester Stallone and Demi Moore through the jungle that is New York real estate. (One actor who worked with Stein supposedly called her "Buddy Hackett with tits.") Andrew was getting rather difficult himself, since he wasn't seeing anything affordable that he liked. But one day the two of them were walking around the Upper East Side when Stein recognized Mike Nichols's secretary coming out of his brownstone and, knowing it was on the market, asked if they could look around. It was perfect. The house had light and atmosphere, room for our furniture and pets, a great space for entertaining. But it was vastly expensive. Andrew cleverly negotiated a deal to rent the house until it was sold, and we finally moved our things out of storage. The day I looked out our street-level kitchen window to see a homeless person going through our garbage, I thought: *I am a New Yorker.*

If I'd known just how steep a learning curve I was about to embark on in negotiating British–American cultural differences, I might never have come. At first, I simply felt that I spoke the same language, I knew New York, I loved American style and was open to getting to grips with anything I didn't know, so what was the big deal? I quickly discovered that American English and English English are not the same language at all, especially with regard to rules of professional etiquette that have never crossed the Atlantic.

193

Misunderstandings started over basic fashion terms. When I talked about "jumpers" or "knickers," the staff would nod at me in frozen incomprehension. (Translation: jumper = sweater; knickers = panties.) What I thought of as ordinary colloquialisms, such as "sacking" and "pinching," required an interpreter (sack = fire; pinch = hire). If I remarked that someone must have "lost a stone" or asked for "the best stalls" at the theater, people would turn pale or crack up with laughter. (Fortunately, my staff quickly learned the latter was always the more appropriate response with me.) I'd ask for a "dummy," a mock-up of the magazine in which pages are pasted as they arrive from the printers. That was unheard of at *Bazaar*. The managing editor and I, two grown-up professional women, were often reduced to sign language or show-and-tell, holding up bits of paper and pointing to whatever the hell it was we were trying to tell each other.

My damned politeness kept getting in the way. To conclude a meeting, I'd say, "Would you like to go away and think about that?" Then I'd sit in my office and wait, but nothing came back. What I expected was what happened at British *Vogue*: People would go to their desks, make some calls, gather their thoughts, and return with a fully fledged idea. I realized that I couldn't make vague noises that sounded like suggestions and had to force myself to command: "Please do this, come here, get that, go there," all of which sound extremely blunt and rude to an English person, even with the "please" thrown in. I was so tentative and civilized with Paul Cavaco that I made him crazy. He'd show me pictures of models and I'd say, "Hmm, I'm not sure about that girl," meaning, in polite English mode, "I don't want to use her." Paul would look at me and tap out another cigarette (he was oblivious to New York's stringent smoking regulations, and his office at the end of a corridor was enveloped in a blue haze). Then he'd inhale and say in his best Bette Davis voice, "Would you please speak American? Do you want her or not? Get off the fucking fence." And I'd shriek, "I'm not on the fence! *I don't want her!*"

Which was fine too. Because I thought of my senior staff as creative peers, we quickly established an easy modus operandi that

194

meant we could have adult discussions, but be as churlish and trivial and insulting to each other as we liked. *Bazaar* has a friendly, almost family atmosphere, which is the way I think it should be in a business where work and leisure blend inextricably together and where there are heavy demands on people's private lives. A lot of New York editors, whatever their nationality, had tough reputations, and since word had got around about how strictly *Vogue* was run, people figured that was the British way of doing things. I wanted *Bazaar* to be a creative and happy place, where people are dedicated to generating the most original and exciting pages and aren't paralyzed by fear, intrigue, back-stabbing, and the strain of working unreasonable hours.

While I was off promoting the magazine, the managing editor, Marguerite Kramer, shouldered the organizational responsibility, but she was so anxious, she'd become a slavedriver. People were working until two A.M., going home for a few hours' sleep, and dragging back to their desks at eight the next morning—weekends too. When I found out, I was furious. I took Marguerite into my office and closed the door.

"You can't work these people so hard," I said.

She looked astonished. "Oh," she said, "I assumed this was what you wanted." Marguerite became a trusted colleague after I got her to lighten up and to convey to the staff that they could be efficient without driving themselves into the ground.

ONE OF MY major adjustments was having to sort through the avalanche of invitations to dinners, cocktail parties, auctions, and balls that began to arrive on my desk. There's a circuit of charitable fund-raisers in New York, many more than in London, where good work is done and my presence was expected, at a Hearst-underwritten table. Literacy, landmark preservation, nature conservancy, various legal defense funds, the opera, the ballet, the museums, and every disease known to man- or womankind—each organization or cause picks an honorary chair who will draw a monied crowd, the women in their best couture. Sometimes it's entertaining, sometimes not.

All these social engagements, and the requests for interviews that heated up as we got closer to the September launch, made me realize that I would need public relations advice, someone to sort through the solicitations and manage publicity about *Bazaar*. Hiring Susan Magrino was my first big step away from British protocol. As I signed her contract, I thought of Beatrix Miller, who believed that one's name should be in the papers three times in life: birth, marriage, and death. I thought of my London friends chorusing, "Who does she think she is?"

As the editor of a British magazine, I was seldom called upon to make speeches or television appearances—it just wasn't done—but in New York, scarcely a day went by that I didn't get a request to go on *New York 1* or *Good Morning America*, to address a group of women executives, or to host one of those charity functions. If I was going to be taken seriously, I had to learn to speak effectively, and I had the feeling that people were paying attention to my British accent, not to my substance. I met with the renowned speech and image consultant Dorothy Sarnoff, who coaches politicians and newscasters in a room that's set up with cameras like a sound studio. She tried to teach me how to modulate my staccato speech, how to breathe, how to chant to myself "I'm glad I'm here, I'm glad you're here" before every speech or interview. I wasn't learning anything that couldn't be summed up in the words "Slow down and relax," but I was willing to consider the advice, until we got to *my* territory: clothes. The conventional wisdom for appearing on-camera dictates a red suit with a scarf tied at the neck and pinned with a brooch, hair teased and sprayed into place. I listened and thought: Nobody tells *me* how to dress. I tell *other* people how to dress. I'm the editor-in-chief of *Harper's Bazaar*, I wear black, and my hair falls where it will.

Susan Magrino was a drill sergeant, trying to eradicate my casual Britishisms and golly-gee naïveté. "Never let me hear you say the word 'jolly' again!" she chided. Instead of deflecting a compliment with British self-deprecation, I was trained to respond with a gracious "Thank you." It was like learning a foreign language. We're not allowed to be fabulous in England, and the word "ambitious" is an insult. Americans are not coy about achievement, and I began to find that liberating. Susan got apoplectic only once, just before the launch of the September issue in late August. I was exhausted, my parents were coming for a visit, and we'd rented a house in the Hamptons for a brief respite at the end of the summer. "What do you mean, 'going to the country with Mummy and Daddy'?" she screamed. "How am I going to reach you? Do you have a phone? A fax? An answering machine? Call waiting? What do I use, a post office box?" That was the last time I was ever so English about telecommunications. I finally got the full import of the high-stakes game we were playing. The curiosity and anticipation became so extreme that Susan was offered a bribe to release an advance copy of the magazine, which was strictly embargoed until its official publication date. We even had to send extra security to guard the printing plant in Kentucky. Everyone was waiting to see if *Bazaar* was any good, if we could we cut it.

We didn't know ourselves. Before the magazine was bound, the final page proofs came to the office, and the impact of the whole could be seen for the first time. Fabien and Marguerite put the pages in a brown paper package and drove at warp speed to the beach house so we could all look at them together. We assembled the pages ourselves. The single coverline next to the model in a Donna Karan black beaded bodysuit was both an announcement and an invitation: "Enter the Era of Elegance," and the word "Bazaar" was playfully nudged atilt by her graceful upturned wrist. For the first time, we could see the full power of Fabien's design and typography. It looked like nothing else in the world. It used space with such a deft, airy grace that the letter *Q*, at the beginning of "Quiet Luxury" in the opening fashion pages, was enough to make you linger for minutes. Christy Turlington looked like a movie queen from a time, as Norma Desmond put it, when stars had faces, but the clothes were modern, streamlined, and totally accessible. There was Kate Moss (in her first American fashion magazine spread) in edgy, funky photographs portraying a baby

197

doll, a hippie chick, a ragamuffin, a buccaneer. The features were as enticing as the fashion: Brooke Shields in her journalistic debut writing about Marguerite Duras, and Jean-Jacques Annaud, the director of the film based on Duras's novel *The Lover*, writing about being on location in Vietnam. There were articles on multicultural education and the neglect of women in medical research. (Did *you* know that the first studies about breast cancer were done on *men?*) Page by page, our spirits rose. The magazine looked strong, thick with advertising from all the designers who had pledged confidence.

Perhaps the most satisfying part was the chance to thumb my nose at the skeptics and naysayers. When I left British *Vogue* amid dire predictions of "you'll never eat lunch in this town again," one of my former colleagues, speaking anonymously in the London *Sunday Times*, said, "Liz will find all the supermodels booked. Linda Evangelista for a cover? No way."

The model in the beaded bodysuit on my first *Harper's Bazaar* cover was Linda Evangelista.

# 13

I ONCE HEARD a hairdresser comment that he had never given a permanent haircut. I feel similarly about magazines. Certainly we tried to make the first and every subsequent issue of *Harper's Bazaar* perfect—elegant and exciting, with a more graceful, grown-up pace than I saw in the competition—but the wonderful thing about my work is that every four weeks there's another issue to play with, another chance to improve. A magazine is meant to change and evolve, particularly with a mercurial subject like fashion.

My first issue of *Bazaar* coincided with its 125th anniversary, marked by a tribute at Saks Fifth Avenue. The window displays were *tableaux vivants*, with live models enacting office meetings and studio sittings, including a faux Liz Tilberis in a white wig. That celebration, combined with newsstand sales of nearly twice the number of the preceding issue's, and advertising pages doubled from the same time the previous year, made for a gratifying month. People *got* us. But not everyone. Some snipers (naturally unattributed) in *Women's Wear Daily* carped that the magazine was too retro. I knew I couldn't please the world. All I can say is that we intended to remind the readers of *Bazaar*'s glorious past as a standard of excellence, to forge a new identity by evoking an illustrious heritage. And within a few months, it was clear that imitation was the sincerest form of flattery. Fabien Baron's floating, candy-colored, overlapping graphics were copied immediately in other publications, advertising campaigns, TV commercials, and packaging. Seeing such mimicry, usually done badly, made us laugh. No point in getting litigious—it meant we were hot.

The most important review was the National Magazine Awards. The American Society of Magazine Editors gives out its Ellies at a luncheon every spring at the Waldorf-Astoria that is like an industry bar mitzvah, and there is great secrecy and speculation about the winners. "Don't expect too much," Claeys Bahrenburg had told me. "This is an intellectual community. Fashion magazines don't win." The first category in which we were nominated was design. As the nominees were being announced, our art director, Joel Berg, happened to look up and notice the overhead lights swiveling toward our table. "I think we've won," he whispered, and moments later, Fabien Baron's name was announced, amid tremendous whooping from our crowd. When it came time for the photography award, Joel was glancing up again. "Don't look now," he said, "but the lights are back." As *Bazaar* was pronounced the winner, Claeys jumped up and punched the air, yelling, "Yesss!" Fabien and I rode back to the office together, screaming all the way and waving our Ellies out the window.

I DON'T KNOW whether the world of fashion magazines is exponentially more deranged than, say, investment banking or air-traffic controlling or supervising a maximum-security prison. You be the judge—eavesdrop on a typical day:

A meeting for the September 1997 issue: I'm with Tonne Goodman and the fashion team gathered around corkboards pinned with hundreds of Polaroids, each tagged with a yellow Post-it, showing the new fall clothes. A collapsible armless muslin dummy is hanging from a hook like a Virginia ham to display the clothes we want to see.

"Pull down the majors. Okay, so it's Prada, Jil, Donna with her sheerness under there."

"You want the little tiny purity one."

"Is Versace in 'Must Haves'?"

"No, we don't have those beaded things."

"He had a ton of black leather."

"Do I need a Valentino if the others are not doing it?"

"There's no Versace in the leather story. Why did she think there was?"

"She loved it."

"I don't think it's anything to do with love. With a white shirt, that would be all right. It's not uncute."

"I think that's Elvis territory."

"This is more 'Day for Night,' because it's velvet."

"This wasn't our first choice, but we're stuck with it."

"Are we just bored with this altogether?"

"Take a look at that gray coat—an ugliness you can't even describe."

"Did they do a tuxedo? Because they do those pretty well."

"I was thinking of doing the leather shirt in the 'Must Haves.' It's kind of sexy."

"We'll get a guilty conscience and then put him in."

"Do we really care about this?"

"Do we have Tyler somewhere?"

"Those purple shoes are so entertaining to look at."

"This is your camisole. This is your 'Chunky.' This is your Ralph."

"Or a chic felted cashmere shirt. Can I sell that to you?"

"He does the most beautiful long gray evening dress—can you go in that direction?"

"But my beading has got to be Mr. Armani."

"The evening suit is Yohji."

"Kristen doesn't wear fur."

"She's going to have to."

"I was thinking of doing a fur that's recycled or fake. Will Amber wear recycled fur?"

"Let's take these off because they're so depressing."

"Are you using the one with the tulle?"

"Maybe the little Isaac suit—makes a great picture."

"Is there anybody in Paris we're losing?"

"Dior was handled in leather. Givenchy . . ."

"Oh, Gucci."

"Chanel had those long wrapover coats."

"You know, some of that collection wasn't made up—it's crucifying."

"So. Oscar. In coats. The lace was Oskie."

"Are you going to take a lot of white shirts?"

"I'd love to, if that's the way you want me to handle it."

"Am I missing 'The Trouser'?"

"The slouch as a story—you've already done so much of it."

"This is Heavy Glamour."

On to a budget meeting in my office. Managing editor Karen Johnston (who joined the magazine in 1995) is tallying how much we've spent on sittings for the current issue and is trying to remind the fashion editors that while we're not holding any telethons for the Hearst family, they'd probably like to retain some of the family fortune rather than paying for the excesses of pampered models and photographers on location:

"That sitting was budgeted at twenty thousand and came in at thirty-six."

"He's not even one of the expensive ones. You eat cheese sandwiches with him and stay at motels."

" 'Navy and White' was thirty-one thousand. There's a seven-thousand-dollar location fee built into that—we were all furious about it."

"Somebody might want to shoot in the Bronx Zoo, but if it costs seven thousand a day, Just Say No. And you might want to rethink the Plaza Athenée, where it costs twenty-five hundred just to get in the door."

"Remember the bill from Industria, where they kept ordering espressos and carrot juice?"

"I remember the days when we had a hot plate and a box of Quik."

"How do you handle telephone and laundry?"

"Have the hotel give them a letter when they check in: 'Your room and tax is paid. The mini-bar is not. Room service for dinner only.'"

"If they want to have room service because it's a late, rainy night . . ."

"Her bill had massages, video rentals, plus dinner for twelve of her friends."

"You have to take some responsibility for the overage. If it goes through, can't you un-charge it against the bill?"

"We're flying the model first class. You guys don't get that."

"These girls have so much mileage. We should say, 'We're happy to pay business class, and you can use miles to upgrade.'"

"This is a reflection of the times. Everybody's doing the same thing. We have to stick our neck out."

"We're going to have a purge. There is a purge in progress."

"Some of them are spoiled brats. And the agents pander, they're so afraid of losing them."

"How about four hundred rolls of film for an eight-page sitting? They're supposed to use five rolls per shot."

"We don't even get the unused part returned. They just put a little bit in the fridge."

"Whisk them in to see me next time they're in the office. I can be as rude as the next person."

"It's getting as cheap here as Italian *Vogue*."

"Well, hello, welcome to the real world."


SUCH RAILLERY GOES with my informal way of working. I put a white shabby-chic sofa in my office so that it's a welcoming place for the staff to hang out, drink coffee, do postmortems on the previous night's activities, and bounce around ideas. Even though it requires enormous discipline to churn out the magazine every month, we're pretty relaxed when we're not on deadline. I might be having an intense consultation with Annemarie Iverson, the beauty and fashion news director, about the precise color of nail polish we must have on our toes now. Richard Sinnott, the accessories director, might arrive with Polaroids of the current essential six-inch stilettos, modeled by himself. I love all this: How could I not? Just because fashion is a multibillion-dollar industry doesn't mean you can't have fun.

When I first arrived at *Bazaar*, I received a note (composed on an antique typewriter, judging by the rickety print) from Helen Gurley Brown, the longtime editor of *Cosmopolitan*, another Hearst publication. "Come and see me when you have time," she wrote. One day I went to her office. It was like walking into a wonderful old drawing, or a Barbara Cartland novel, all pink and floral and needlepointed, the sort of room where a Victorian heroine fell onto a chaise longue holding a hankie because her soldier boy had gone to war. Helen was cordial and flattering. Then she got to her point. "What sort of coverlines are you going to use?" she asked, and I realized she wanted to ensure that she wouldn't have any competition in the "Ten Ways to Have an Out-of-Body Orgasm" department. Some time later she sent me another little note about a wigmaker who made hairpieces for the crotch. The story wasn't right for *Cosmo*, but she wondered if I'd like it for *Bazaar*.

No, I'm not interested in pubic wigmakers. But features are particularly tricky for a magazine like *Bazaar*, as witnessed by the fact that I went through three different editors before importing Eve MacSweeney as features director, who'd done such a terrific job at British *Vogue*. Our stories must be fearless, sophisticated, irreverent, sexy, unpredictable, their taste and sensibilities complementing the fashion content. I don't want to wait for a trend to be established—I'm happy to make people sit up and take notice for the first time. Alongside cutting-edge art and design stories, Hollywood profiles and thought-provoking essays, we've covered such subjects as Anita Hill, Madeleine Albright, Joycelyn Elders,

Marian Wright Edelman, girl gangs, lesbian mothers, domestic violence among the gentry, child labor in Pakistan, women on death row. Sometimes these stories create controversy. We got a lot of flak for an article about the erotic life of Islamic women. This sort of reaction confounds me. *Of course* Muslims must have an erotic life, or there wouldn't be any new Muslims. Hello?

Probably the hardest decision to make every month is what to put on the cover, which is much more than a pretty picture of a pretty girl. A cover has to seduce the woman in the street, making the magazine walk off the newsstand by itself. The coverlines are carefully thought out: not too patronizing or highbrow, not too off-putting. We want the reader to think: *Hmmm*. There is no formula for the picture, but in general a smile is better than a frown, warm is better than cold, full face is better than profile, a direct gaze is better than averted eyes. Too pretty doesn't sell well; a little aggressiveness does. A style that's reminiscent of Veronica Lake might work inside the magazine, but the cover should be fairly modern. We're looking for something simmering, assertive, something about the twist of the lip, the length of the neck, a beautiful face on a clean, strong, white background. When the pictures from a cover sitting come in, the best ones will jump out, and they're posted on a wall of the art department. (Fabien and his staff used to throw darts at them, until the wall was filled with so many holes it had to be replastered.) Sometimes a photograph never intended to be a cover comes in with a wonderful graphic feel, and the girl is looking straight at the camera, sexy and smiling, and we know that's it, but mostly we plan more carefully than that. Babies and men have certain curb appeal, but we have to be careful to keep the fashion content uppermost.

There are services that do "market research" about covers, asking potential readers hypothetical questions to gauge their preferences ("Would you like this model to be your friend? Would you like to have her lip gloss? Would you like her to be holding a kitten?"). But I've always been suspicious that the people used for research don't reflect the demographic of our readers. Once, while still at British *Vogue*, I was having curtains made by a lovely lady who came from a town called Lincoln and probably had not bought any new clothes since the end of World War II. "You know, luv," she said in her North Country accent as she was measuring the windows, "I'm one of those people in the market research for *Vogue*." I realized that it was her yea or nay on a questionnaire that was running my magazine.

I've had to acknowledge that celebrity sells in America, even though an actress is not a professional model, and we don't always get what we want. It's useful to put stars on the covers of traditionally slimmer issues, those between-seasons summer months when there aren't any new clothes in the stores. Sharon Stone and Drew Barrymore don't sell *Bazaar* particularly well, but Madonna and Demi Moore do—go figure. If we're doing a tie-in with a film, we try to make sure it's a good one. Winona Ryder and Daniel Day-Lewis made a powerful cover around the time of *The Crucible*. If our cover model has been in the *National Enquirer* the week before, I know we'll sell big. When Patrick Demarchelier shot the cover of Elizabeth Hurley and Hugh Grant with a chimpanzee, he kept enthusing, "Divine!"—forgetting that it was a hooker named Divine who had just gotten Grant in trouble. That cover was one of our bestsellers, along with Courtney Love and the two issues featuring the Princess of Wales.

Our special projects editor, Maggie Buckley, is a genius at handling the tyranny of celebrities photographed for the cover or for fashion sittings. (Maggie came from American *Vogue*. When she told Anna Wintour she was leaving, Anna said, "No, you're not." And when Maggie insisted that yes, she was, Anna paused and, in her best what-I-say-goes mode, said, "Let me think about it.") Maggie is the person who deals with the layers of nightmare publicists and managers, who has to tell the Artist Formerly Known as Prince, "No, you cannot have your personal retoucher fly in from Minneapolis to tidy up the photos." Sometimes it's hard to remember that celebrities are just as insecure as the rest of us, maybe more so. When we did a sitting with Val Kilmer, he kept calling me to ask was it a good idea, and what should he wear, and was the photographer talented, and on and on. "Do you have a piano?" I finally asked. He did. "You are going to put these pictures on the piano for the rest of your life," I said. That did the trick. But I missed the best celebrity sitting of all: We were going to be shooting Aretha Franklin, and I suggested that a piano be put in the studio. She entertained the troops all day long while being photographed.

The task that I love best and traditionally save for myself, no matter how frenetic my schedule, is assembling the photo spreads on the fashion shows: pret-a-porter in London, Milan, and Paris in March and October, then the New York collections in April and November, and the ne plus ultra, Paris couture in January and July. The shows are like a traveling circus—hundreds and hundreds of magazine and newspaper editors, television reporters, still photographers, store executives, buyers, and celebrity clients gather en masse dozens of times during Fashion Week, squeezing into a tent or a loft or a theater to see the lavish excesses of each designer's mind. When the shows started to become productions worthy of Cecil B. DeMille, new venues had to be found. Now the collections may be shown in the basement of the Louvre or at a covered-over hotel swimming pool. The Givenchy couture collection by Alexander McQueen in summer 1997 was presented at a Byzantine hospital where corpses were once dissected for medical research, and Chanel showed under a plastic tent at the Musée Rodin. The temperature rose to about 120 degrees, and Suzy Menkes, the fashion editor of the *International Herald Tribune*, fainted in the heat, as she often does.

The shows are also a tough time for the models, who must register at their hotels under pseudonyms and scurry out back doors two steps ahead of their groupies, male and female. I remember Bridget Hall dropping signed photographs out the window of the Four Seasons Hotel down to the street for screaming fans.

Grace Coddington and I always arrange for adjoining seats on the same overnight flight to Europe—we refer to this as "sleeping with the enemy." I always stay in the same room on the fourth floor of the Ritz, with long French windows facing south. The designers send wonderful flower arrangements, and I become a

207

horticulturist, tending to my garden every day. I feel like a movie star, even though I take only two suitcases of clothes and very little jewelry.

Often we pay visits to the design studios before a show, when the models are having their fittings and the designer's whole atelier—from the fabric cutters to the "suits," the business backers—is in high gear, and we get to touch and examine the clothes, even render an opinion. The designer might ask, "What do you think?" and we'll say, "How about pink gloves with that, or pink hair?" On the day of the show, sketches or photos of each complete outfit are pinned up in the dressing room as visual cues, and there are signs on the wall articulating the designer's wishes about creating a mood as the girls go out on the runway: DON'T SMILE OR LOOK STRAIGHT AHEAD OR WALK FASTER.

Getting inside the show is a scene from *Day of the Locust*, with poseurs trying to finesse their way past the bullies guarding the gate, and swarms of bodies jockeying for space. (I've only had to punch a security guard that one time.) Inside, ushers called "red ties" are assigned to run interference for us and find our seats. Once when I was struggling to enter a show from a crowded Paris sidewalk, the mob suddenly parted like the Red Sea and I walked in with my team. This is when I knew I had a powerful job.

I'm not particularly claustrophobic. I've dutifully braved the crush of people, snaking electrical wires, rickety steps, lack of air. But on one occasion we were supposed to attend a dinner after a show in the courtyard of an old castle that had been covered over with scaffolding and a tarp. Everything looked beautiful—white tablecloths, red roses—but it started to rain, and waiters were trying to disperse the puddles on the makeshift roof by poking at it with long poles. I took one look and said, "I'm not going in there." We left shortly before the scaffolding and tarp collapsed, sending water and steel cascading over the guests. Fortunately, only one person was slightly injured.

I was flying the Concorde to Paris, sitting next to Rose Marie Bravo, who was until recently the president of Saks Fifth Avenue and is now CEO of Burberrys, plus a whole flock of other fashion folk. Our shrimp cocktails had just been placed in front of us when we heard a noise like a bomb, and the plane started to dive. There was no smoke, no smell, no screaming, no announcement from the pilot. We just dipped about 20,000 feet, the serving carts rolling down the aisle. Rose Marie and I clutched hands, assuming we were about to die. After what seemed like an eternity, the plane leveled off. One of the passengers rushed up to the cockpit and came back to report that the Concorde, which normally travels at supersonic speed, had gone subsonic in one engine. We returned to New York, crawling and bumping the whole way. Rose Marie told me that in those few desperate moments, she thought: *Liz can't die—she's a mother.* But, undeterred, all the fashion near-victims got on the next Air France Concorde, where the crew broke out the champagne and caviar; we arrived in Paris at four A.M.

Most fashion adventures are not so dramatic, more a matter of some slight, real or perceived, to a fragile or inflated ego. Alleged grown-ups turn into grammar-school children over who's assigned to the first row at a show or who gets to sit next to Sting. In the summer of 1997, at the same time that Demi Moore was on the cover of *Harper's Bazaar*, she joined us at the couture shows, provocatively standing right in front of Anna Wintour and asking in a stage whisper, "Where is my seat? Oh, there's Liz, it must be next to her." When she was late for a dinner party at Karl Lagerfeld's, Karl kept asking me, "When does Hollywood arrive?" People critique, gossip, and check one another out until the lights go down—designers are notoriously unpunctual. (Joan Juliet Buck, the editor of French *Vogue*, once declared she would walk out on any show that started more than fifteen minutes late, but her remonstrance didn't last long—the designers have recourse by pulling their advertising.) The music comes up, there is a tremendous flashing of lightbulbs, and it's all over rather quickly. Every show used to end with a fantasy bridal gown as a coda for the collection, but sadly that happens less now. Then we pile in a car, and it's on to the next show. The driver is the most important person in the pack. Between shows he gets us ham sandwiches to eat in the car while we discuss, trash, ridicule, and admire what we just saw. And if I'm leaving Gucci on my way to Armani, I might change my jacket in the back seat. My husband went to one fashion show and swore he'd never go to another. Frankly, he couldn't care less about the swish of clothes or swish of people (although he is my severest critic—sometimes when we are in separate cities, I'll call and describe my outfit, so accustomed am I to soliciting his approval).

I've worked with designers for a quarter of a century, and I find most of them to be great characters. I especially love the glimpses I get of their exquisite homes, like Valentino's seventeenth-century gabled red brick chateau outside Paris. There are two box-hedged flower gardens—one for admiring, one for cutting—and as you turn the corner and come out of the forest, the deer and rabbits scatter. Behind the chateau is a huge lawn with ancient yew trees that look like ladies in crinoline skirts.

Parties after a show, when the designer can relax after months of work, are like family affairs, with friends and lovers, dogs and cats, even ghosts: At lunch in the atelier after a Christian Lacroix show, his business partner Jean-Jacques Picard looked at me and suddenly rushed out of the room, claiming he'd seen the ghost of a dark-haired woman hovering over my head. (Personally, I think it was Andrew's mother.) Tom Ford, the designer who resuscitated Gucci, has a beautiful Paris apartment with a Jack Russell terrier named John who is an exhibitionist: During one dinner, John sat with his legs wide apart, licking himself. (I now leave risqué messages for John on Tom's answering machine.) Before Versace's death, all the models in his show would wear their favorite dresses from the collection to dinner at Gianni's Milan palazzo, making a grand entrance past the marble pilasters, bas reliefs, bronze figurines, Picassos, and Warhols. At one such dinner, the magician David Copperfield surreptitiously walked around the tables, set with more gold than any royalty would expect, and switched placecards so he could sit next to Claudia Schiffer, later his betrothed. At one Versace couture dinner, I had the best time of all, sitting with Elton John and Lisa Marie Presley.

"When I was a little girl," Lisa Marie told Elton, "I told my father I liked your music, and he bought me your trilogy album." Elton almost turned blue. "You mean Elvis Presley bought one of my albums?" he asked with awe.

"Yeah," she answered, "but I think he was kind of hurt that I didn't ask for *his* music."

Flying my senior staff to Europe for the pret-a-porter collections, feeding them, and lodging them costs $100,000, an admittedly exorbitant sum, but these shows are absolutely necessary for our work. As we sit and sketch, we are building a library of information for the next six months' issues; it's a biannual shot of vitality. Outside the industry, fashion shows may seem extravagant and extreme, and sometimes they are. (At a 1997 Valentino show, with its models styled as Siberian warriors, John Fairchild, the former publisher of *Women's Wear Daily*, turned to me and said, "These women eat their young.") As for couture, it's the last bastion of a historic tradition of tailoring and dressmaking, and its standards of excellence cannot be replicated for mass consumption. But it has a huge power to enliven and stimulate. Pret-a-porter is more limited in its flights of fancy because these clothes have to *sell*, but it can be equally inspirational as its messages are filtered down. Runway fantasy must become retail reality. At every price point, we all absorb the designers' latest impulses. The distance from Karl Lagerfeld to Kmart is shorter than you might imagine.

ONE DAY, I was walking along Fifty-fourth Street to lunch when I saw a man washing a store awning. I stood and watched for a few minutes as each section of canvas became a perfect cornflower blue under his cloth. Sometimes I wish I had a job like that, with a clear beginning, middle, and end. In fashion, we're constantly trying to reinvent the wheel in images that generate excitement. It ain't easy.

The fashion industry, including *Harper's Bazaar*, was the subject of recent opprobrium for promoting what was dubbed "heroin chic," a tag that referred to a new generation of models and photographic styles: raw, hip, harsh, stripped of pretense; the models with lanky hair, stringbean bodies, and moody expressions. It was fashion redefining itself, endorsing an untraditional kind of glamour and beauty, much as it had done in the 1960s. But there was a backlash. The controversy reached critical mass in February 1997 when Davide Sorrenti, a twenty-year-old photographer, died of a heroin overdose. (His brother Mario, also a photographer who often works for *Bazaar*, shot the famous Calvin Klein Obsession campaign featuring his girlfriend at the time, Kate Moss.) Davide's death stirred up the whole hornet's nest of drug use and imagery in fashion. There were a lot of Monday-morning quarterbacks after the event, with modeling agents blaming photographers and art directors for their complicity in creating images that seemed to endorse dangerous behavior, and editorial staffs blaming the agents for failing to monitor their young charges. President Clinton himself admonished the industry to clean up its act.

Some of the images that were published in *Detour* and the British magazine *I-D* and in some advertising campaigns did, to my way of thinking, breach the boundaries of taste and responsibility. Although *Bazaar* was accused by some of espousing heroin chic, I would certainly never have permitted pictures with explicitly druggy overtones to be published in the magazine, and must agree to disagree with those who say otherwise. But the reason this is such a complicated and contentious subject is that there is a fine line between imparting appropriate messages and pushing the envelope of art—and what we do every month is nothing less than fashion as art. Looking at exquisite, often expensive clothes in a magazine is akin to seeing paintings in a museum: You can enjoy the beauty and talent, even though you're not going to take them home and make them part of your life. All of us have shelvesful of beloved J. Crew sweats, but there is no point in creating a fashion magazine that is indistinguishable from a J. Crew catalog. We provide the dreams alongside the reality of fashion.

If fashion is sometimes controversial, sometimes difficult to absorb, it is only a matter of time before it works its way to acceptability: A slip dress that at first seems too revealing is deemed utterly demure next season, even with bra straps showing. A fur coat, considered abhorrent one winter, becomes all the rage the next. We enjoy the process of reinventing ourselves, the opportunity to see ourselves in different lights. When we first saw grunge from Anna Sui and Marc Jacobs at Perry Ellis in 1992, it wasn't attractive, but it was young, cool, and gritty. As reporters, we can't ignore or dismiss anything fashion offers. Fashion is about change, fantasy, whimsy, reassessment. *Life* is about choices, and we make choices about clothes just as we do in other arenas of our lives. Fashion can accommodate a spectrum of choices, even within one closet, where it seems perfectly reasonable to hang a skintight, show-me-those-abs Gucci dress next to an extra-large Gap sweatshirt.

Fashion is a reflecting pool of the wider world, its impulses and its self-doubt about those impulses. There *is* a serious drug problem among a small percentage of models and photographers, as there is in the rest of society and as there has always been through the years—only the drug of choice has changed since the days when I detected the odor of rotten eggs at a sitting. Many of the girls come from small towns, and are unsophisticated and inexperienced, full of youthful assumptions of immortality and vulnerable to predators within and without the business. Some model agents are honorable and avuncular, some are unscrupulous and mercenary, with no real concern about the welfare of their wards, who are so replaceable. (They'll eventually be replaced even if they stay clean and sober.)

We know a lot of secrets that we handle with utter discretion because people have problems and private lives. Only when I am rocking on the porch of my retirement home will I name names— my mother raised no stupid children. We know who is sleeping with whom, and who is not sleeping with whom. We know which models have gone into rehab and which ones should be admitted PDQ. We are not in the "outing" business. We certainly care about drug abuse and should be partners with model agencies in insisting that it will not be tolerated. But a model can be strung out in the sunniest sort of photographs. And the truth is that the moment is over for the somber mood that could, at its most extreme, be

213

called heroin chic. We've already moved on, not necessarily for benevolent reasons but because fashion always moves on, too fast and free to be motivated by political correctness. As I write this, there are lots of smiles, not frowns or blank stares, in the photos we're producing, and the paradigm of the new model is a more generously proportioned, classically pretty, American Beauty. The edge and angst of recent times is gone. Even Kate Moss is starting to look like Grace Kelly.

But we're always making *somebody* mad, the latest outrage being computer enhancement of photographs. With modern technology, we can elongate torsos, eliminate freckles, or change the color of a dress. When a cover photo of Princess Caroline revealed slightly mottled pigmentation, a snippet of flawless skin from another photograph was patched in, and voilà—a milkmaid's complexion. For the September 1997 cover of Courtney Love, our art director, Paul Eustace, fixed what looked like a stump at the end of her knee because her legs were tucked under, superimposing a leg from another picture. It's like plastic surgery performed by the art department. Magazines have been doing such touch-ups for years—Cindy Crawford's mole was routinely airbrushed out and many a celebrity has had wrinkles zapped. The computer now allows almost any kind of change imaginable, but we use it infrequently and judiciously. Is it deceptive? I don't think so, no more than push-up bras, orthodontia, mascara, and undereye concealer.

Now I'll tell you what makes *me* mad: designers whose ego overtakes their talent, models who start to believe their own press, fashion reporters who just don't get it, jewelry manufacturers who are insulted when we photograph their wares on urban Hispanics, the merchandising of product lines that have nothing to do with a designer's skills, and the person at the American Society of Magazine Editors who denied *Bazaar* another award, saying we had broken the rule about separation of editorial and advertising content with the black background of a Calvin Klein ad that coincidentally looked like it seeped over to the jagged edge of a fashion story on the facing page.

MY JOB GETS me invited to a lot of interesting places. The scope of social opportunity when I arrived at *Bazaar* was stunning— Britain is much more cliquish, and the editor of a fashion magazine doesn't automatically socialize with politicians, authors, sports figures, architects. From a background of zips-and-hems, I was now dining at the apartment of Veronica and Randolph Hearst in a room painted like the Bois de Boulogne, with Boutros Boutros-Ghali, Madame Pompidou, and the Aga Khan as my fellow guests. At one Hearst party, I listened in while Carolyn Bessette Kennedy described to Hillary Rodham Clinton her dilemma when she was looking for a book at Barnes & Noble and suddenly found herself in the section on pregnancy. Sure that a tabloid photographer would be lying in wait and would presume that he had stumbled onto a secret, she didn't know whether to bolt, back out quietly, or sit down and weep.

Joe Armstrong, who was consulting with Claeys Bahrenburg on the magazine publishing side at Hearst, was a good friend of Jacqueline Onassis, then a book editor at Doubleday, and arranged for the three of us to have lunch at the Four Seasons in March 1993. As I walked up the broad staircase into the sleek, modern room designed by Philip Johnson, I resisted the temptation to stop at every table and say, "Guess who I'm meeting?" I wanted the whole world to see us together. Instinctively I felt that Mrs. Onassis deserved the same gesture of deference shown to European royals and had to restrain myself from locking one knee into the other for a curtsy when she arrived. She had been a young woman during the glory days of *Harper's Bazaar* and loved the idea that we were resurrecting its flair and elegance. In that distinctive, slightly breathy voice, she asked detailed questions, particularly about photography, which was how she'd earned a living before she was married. I met her on only one other occasion, when she invited me to join her at a benefit for the American Ballet Theater and caused a gasp when she entered the hall in a dress by Carolina Hererra—who was wearing the same dress. The interview I always wanted to get was a dialogue between Mrs. Onassis and the Princess of Wales. I thought they had experienced a similar kind of pressure, being

215

thrust into the limelight by marriage and having to deal with a husband of wandering affections. But it was not to be.

In September 1994 *Harper's Bazaar* underwrote a benefit for the Pediatric AIDS Foundation, the charity started by Elizabeth Glaser, a dynamic woman who lost her seven-year-old daughter to AIDS and was in the last stages of the disease herself, which she'd contracted from blood transfusions during pregnancy and had passed to her daughter through breast milk. The Industria Studio in the meat-packing district of downtown Manhattan was turned into a carnival called Kids 4 Kids, with celebrity entertainers and athletes overseeing the games. Diane Sawyer and Mike Nichols manned a "Gone Fishing" booth, Billy Baldwin and Chynna Phillips were in charge of "Leapfrog," Katie Couric and Tom Brokaw played "Big Mouth Ball-tossing," Kate Moss and Johnny Depp ran the mini-hockey rink, and Michael Douglas spent his fiftieth birthday manning the dunking tank. Andrew and the kids and the whole staff of *Bazaar* and their families came out to work in jeans and white Kids 4 Kids T-shirts. My favorite memento of that day is a photograph of my cochair Donna Karan and me with seven-foot-tall Patrick Ewing, but you can't recognize him because his head is cut off, and our heads are at his waist level. Elizabeth Glaser, desperately ill, had petitioned Hillary Rodham Clinton to be honorary chair of the event, and the First Lady had promised her, "If you get well and come to New York, I'll be there too." Mrs. Clinton brought Chelsea and presented a presidential commendation to Elizabeth, who died just two months later. More than $1 million was raised that day for the Elizabeth Glaser Scientist Award, established to create a corps of the most creative scientific minds in the world to do research in pediatric AIDS.

My children seem to take these celebrity encounters in stride. Trudie Styler, the wife of Sting, organized a concert at Carnegie Hall in April 1995 to benefit the rain forests. In between sets, a man I'd never seen before rushed up to congratulate me. "Your son is interviewing Henry Kissinger in the men's room," he said, impressed. A book had just been published in which Robert McNamara castigated the former secretary of state for his part in the Vietnam War, and Robbie, finding himself standing at the urinals next to Kissinger, decided to find out what he thought about the public reproach. (Kissinger conceded he was embarrassed by McNamara's remarks.)

IN THE FALL of 1994, I was notified that I was to receive a special award from the Council of Fashion Designers of America, and would I please select someone to present it onstage at Lincoln Center in January? I'd been to the CFDA awards the past two years and knew it was incumbent on the honoree to choose a presenter of some esteem and éclat. The first, in fact the only, person I thought of was the Princess of Wales, and I wrote her a note, asking if it would be possible for her to do the honors. Her private secretary at the time, Patrick Jephson, called with her regrets. I still hadn't come up with an alternate a few days later when Jephson called again. "Private secretaries are sometimes very wrong," he said. "The princess would love to come."

I melted to jelly, and then set about planning for the day of her arrival, when I would function as her lady-in-waiting. I suggested British cars to transport her around the city—a Range Rover for day and a Rolls at night. We drove right out onto the tarmac at JFK to pick her up and went straight to a pediatric hospital in Spanish Harlem—I was in charge of holding her handbag so she could hug the children with AIDS. At the luncheon given by Veronica and Randolph Hearst, a white-jacketed waiter stood behind every chair to serve beluga caviar, lamb chops, and mousse. The princess sat next to Ralph Lauren, who asked for her phone number and jokingly offered her a job as a showroom model. "I'll have my office call you," she said amiably.

As Claeys and I waited outside the New York State Theater for the princess, her driver overshot the entrance and I had to run after the car in my black beaded Calvin Klein gown. Diana was wearing a long royal blue sheath designed by Catherine Walker. At her throat was a pearl choker with an egg-size sapphire clasp, a gift from the Queen Mother, and when I remarked on its beauty, she smiled a little wickedly and said, "They're not getting it back either." Her gown was as body-hugging as a bathing suit, with spaghetti straps crossed in back, and she wore her hair slicked back with gel. It was such a sexy and un-princessy look that she appeared in virtually every magazine and on every television newscast around the world. And just off to the side in nearly every shot of her is my mother, who'd come over for the occasion and was also dressed by Calvin Klein. I was too, but Mummy stole the limelight. (On behalf of *Harper's Bazaar*, I tried to buy the princess's dress from that night in the June 1997 charity auction of her clothes at Christie's, but it went for a huge sum, so I settled for another Walker dress in floral-printed chiffon and donated it to the Metropolitan Museum of Art's Costume Institute.)

For our dinner table that night, I'd invited Ralph Lauren, Calvin Klein, Donna Karan, Isaac Mizrahi, and Kate Moss, along with the Hearst executives. Isaac and Kate both wandered in nonchalantly late, by which time I had murder in my heart. So many people came over to talk during dinner that the princess didn't even get to eat, but she was cordial and pleasant with everyone, including my sons, who arrived for the awards ceremony. "Do you guys always wear shirts and ties," she teased, "or is it because you're always coming to see me?" When we left the dinner for the theater to rehearse her entrance, we saw the stage and became absolutely terrified. We then retreated to our seats in the auditorium, where Mummy, Robbie, Chris, and the security guards were having a very lively discussion about the O. J. Simpson case.

We sat in the audience for most of the presentations: Mariah Carey introducing Victor Alfaro, Sigourney Weaver for Richard Tyler, "The Nanny" Fran Drescher for Cynthia Rowley. "Weeellllll," droned Drescher in a voice that sounded like nails on a blackboard, "the Queen of Queens gets to meet the Princess of Wales." We both groaned when Robert Lee Morris accepted an award for his jewelry saying, "Clothing without accessories is like sex without orgasm." Lauren Hutton was wearing a necklace made from New Guinea currency—she said about twenty such pieces would buy a large pig.

Throughout the awards, Diana kept leaning over and whispering, "Shouldn't we be going backstage yet?" Finally we got the sign to prepare for our big moment. A short video was shown in which various designers said such flattering things about me that I kept pinching myself to make sure it wasn't a eulogy. (Isaac Mizrahi said he thought I should be played onscreen by Julie Andrews. He obviously hadn't experienced the lacrosse-stick-wielding, security-guard-punching Liz Tilberis.) Then over the loudspeaker came the announcement, "Ladies and gentlemen, Her Royal Highness, the Princess of Wales." She looked startled and embarrassed by the thundering applause as she walked to the podium, and just as it was quieting down, someone in the audience shouted, "Move to New York!" Diana was still married to Prince Charles, but the papers were full of speculation about the next stage of her life, even suggesting that she might take a job at *Bazaar*. (For the record, I would have cleared an office for her any time she wanted, but we never discussed it.) The princess spoke briefly, but what she said was so lovely: "I am immensely proud to be here in New York tonight with you all to be giving this award to a lady from my own country, who is also a dear friend, and whose talent and courage are an inspiration to us all." As I came out to accept the award, I performed my usual curtsy, kiss on the cheek, and flashed her a smile reserved for and recognized by only those most important in my life. As we walked into the wings, we saw my landlady, Diane Sawyer, who smiled and said generously, "What a couple of stars!"

A theme of the ceremony that night was "Fashion Targets Breast Cancer." Dozens of designers spoke or wrote notes in the program about a mother, daughter, sister, wife, friend, or colleague who had faced the dread disease. I read these tributes and missives feeling grateful and secure myself. I thought cancer was behind me. A few months later, I was to learn I was wrong.

# 14

IT COULDN'T BE happening again is what I was thinking the summer of 1995. Ever since moving to New York, I'd dreamed of these indolent weekends in my own home with my own things (no more guesting or renting) on the eastern end of Long Island—just Andrew and the boys and a few dozen lobsters. We finally bought a house covered in weathered gray shingles and hidden in woods at the edge of a west-facing harbor, abutting an old whaling cemetery. The eclectic furniture collection of the previous owner was still in residence, but we draped my collection of primitive quilts over the banisters and installed the same ten-foot-long pine cupboard we'd taken out of my parents' house and had been transporting to every one of our homes for almost twenty-five years. The boys nailed basketball hoops to every possible surface, indoors and out, and invited friends for family lunches with unalterable menus: Saturday hamburgers out and Sunday roasts in. We'd sit on our deck to watch the sunset, a ball of fire in a mackerel sky, listening to the osprey who'd built her nest atop a telephone pole on our beach and cackled if we came too near her babies ("Mrs.

O," we called her). Biking ten miles a day and returning a serve with an improved backhand, I considered myself healthier than at any time since my twenties. I was feeling and, dammit, even looking good, a solid year beyond the ravages and indignities of hysterectomy and chemotherapy and biopsy. I had put cancer behind me. The only real reminder was my monthly CA–125 blood test. Any number under 35 was considered normal. And in early June, mine hit 193. Somewhere in my body, too infinitesimal to be perceived in any way but this, there was a trace of cancer.

It was a bitter pill, accepting that my body had once more turned against me, but it was not entirely unexpected. Ovarian cancer is like a cockroach, defying an arsenal of poisons. Now we had to call in the big guns, and my doctor did not hesitate for a moment to let me know which of the options available was his heartfelt recommendation: zapping me with megadoses of chemotherapy, followed by bone marrow transplant. BMT: a monogram I was to know as well as my own. Andrew and I tried to listen impassively to Peter Dottino's primer on the subject. "The reason we can't cure cancer is that we can't give enough chemicals without killing the patient," he explained. "The more chemo we give, the worse havoc we wreak." Chemo has a profound effect on bone marrow, the spongy material in the cavities of large bones that's a factory for blood: It makes red cells, which give blood its color and carry oxygen throughout the body; white cells, which fight infection; and platelets, which cause the blood to clot so you don't bleed to death. "BMT allows us to give an essentially lethal treatment and then support the patient," Dottino explained. "We take out some of your own marrow, freeze it in liquid nitrogen, and when you're sicker than shit, we give it back. We haul you to the brink, push you a little bit over, and then pull you back."

BMT was once thought little better than voodoo, so radical that insurance companies waged courtroom battles over covering the costs, but it's now considered frontline defense for some cancer patients. More than 50 percent of those with leukemia are *cured* with the treatment, but it's still unproven against solid tumors like mine. I was given a sheaf of papers blessedly written in English

221

rather than medicalese—the kind of forms that have to pass through many, many hospital committees to ensure that the least sophisticated person in the world knows what she is signing—but there was no mistaking the words "Consent for Research" at the top of every page, and Dottino freely admitted I'd be offering myself up as a guinea pig. I would be only the tenth woman with ovarian cancer to receive this treatment at Mount Sinai, although the National Autologous Bone Marrow Transplant Registry in Milwaukee, Wisconsin, now lists more than 500 women with ovarian cancer from 89 medical centers in North and South America who've been through this procedure. (The reporting is done on a purely voluntary basis, and this figure probably represents only half the actual number who've been treated.)

BMT *sounds* logical: It's like removing the furniture before fumigating the house. But a small number of people die from the remedy itself, and it renders you susceptible to every conceivable kind of complication. Without red cells to carry oxygen, you can become anemic. Without white cells to fight infection, something as simple as athlete's foot can mean big trouble. Without platelets to cause clotting, you can bleed uncontrollably if you cough. I'd be in the hospital, in isolation, for a month. The boys would be in day camp at the beach, Andrew commuting between us, and I didn't know how we would bear to have the family split up. And how could I justify a month off from work?

It is useful to have a doctor in the family at such a time, and when we got home, we sat down at our kitchen table to call my brother, Grant, in what was the middle of the night in England. At first I said flat out, "I'm not going to do it." Grant was in favor of BMT but presented both sides of the argument. I kept circling around the same issue: abandoning the magazine. Andrew spoke with him—I could overhear a one-sided version of the same reasoning—and then handed the phone back to me for the final parry and thrust.

"I don't mean to be brutal," Grant said, "but it's no good worrying about your job, because if you don't have this done, you won't be around to *have* a job." My brother is a considerate and intelligent man. That was enough for me. And I was feeling so well, I frankly expected to sail through it.

I didn't want too much information at first—I'd rather explore the unknown by myself, with Andrew riding shotgun. But I got so much material, from the hospital and from friends who did library and on-line searches, that I became a mini-authority, which is what happens to any informed patient.

Cancer experts don't know exactly why solid tumors are more difficult to vanquish—they respond to chemotherapy, but the cancer often comes back. "It may be that the cells develop resistance to chemo, or inactivate it, or learn how to pump it out as fast as it enters," explained Dr. Edward Trimble of the Cancer Therapy Evaluation Program at the National Cancer Institute. "If we can increase the dose, we can cure more people. With solid tumors, we haven't been able to show that increasing the zapping benefits the patient. But it's most likely to help the woman who has a small volume of cancer left and is sensitive to platinum."

That meant me. I seemed to be the perfect candidate for this harrowing procedure: I had only microscopic cancer in my body, the first cycle of cisplatin having wiped out the rest. On Monday morning I called Dottino, with the tranquillity that comes from having one decision to make and *making* it.

"I'm going for it," I said.

I could hear the energy in his voice. "Come over right *now*," he ordered. But I was not to see much more of him for a while. At the hospital, he handed me off to a new team: the head of the BMT unit, Dr. Steven Fruchtman, and his associate, Dr. Luis Isola; their nurse, Virginia Ross; and social worker Donna Siegal. Dottino yanked Fruchtman out of a meeting to test my marrow right then and there. It was all so sudden, I didn't even have time to get anxious. Dr. Fruchtman was kind and pleasant, and I'm not obsequious to doctors, so I read him the riot act. "You have it within your province not to hurt me," I said, "and if you do, I'm going to scream loud enough to summon the fire brigade." He injected a large dose of numbing medication in my buttocks and pulled a sample of bone marrow out of my hip.

Fruchtman kept trying to make me *think* about the gamble I was taking, evidently believing that an informed patient would be a successful one. "Have you read all the material?" he asked. "Do you have any questions? *Why* don't you have any questions?"

I did have one. "Are you going to kill me?" I asked.

"I'll try not to," he said.

I still had several hurdles to clear: There was a battery of tests for my heart, lungs, and liver to see whether I could withstand the procedure. I had to be physically fit before they almost killed me. And there was the business of convincing my insurance company to pay for it. So many women in my situation find themselves in prolonged battles with managed-care systems. I have heard about HMOs that deny not only state-of-the-art treatment but access to gynecological oncologists and tests important to diagnosis and follow-up care. If you're a cynic, it doesn't take much to make you infer that the insurers are stalling in hopes that a woman will become too ill or too dead to continue fighting. I was lucky, with the help of one Angelina Corsun, a.k.a. Donna Quixote, who argues for insurance coverage on behalf of Mount Sinai patients, tilting at windmills to explain the what, where, and how of new procedures. Insurance companies have maintained that BMT is technically experimental, and they're less than enthusiastic about a $100,000 experiment. One ovarian cancer patient in Sacramento, California, got approval for BMT only after a television reporter doing a program on HMO horror stories contacted the woman's insurer for a response. Other insurers are trying to find a reasonable way to deal with the enormous, potentially lifesaving expense, relying on experts outside their own medical staff to recommend the best candidates for the procedure to try to identify a standard of care. Corsun succeeds in convincing them about 98 percent of the time. And so she did with my case.

With some cancers, like leukemia, the bone marrow itself is compromised by disease, and the transplant must come from a donor, preferably a brother or sister, since you are most genetically similar to a sibling. (Each of your parents contributes only half of your genes.) But I was eligible for an autologous transplant, storing a batch of my own marrow—just like you can now donate your own blood before surgery—in a procedure called harvesting. Botanical terms seemed to crop up: I was told that putting marrow back after chemo is like planting seeds in a garden and hoping they grow in the scorched earth. It also reminded me of yogurt starter.

Skipping the couture shows, I was scheduled for the harvest right after the Fourth of July, thinking all weekend that it was a good thing I'm "the enemy" and didn't have a patriotic holiday ruined. I was surprisingly cool, even eager. If I have a problem and someone offers a solution, I'm satisfied and grateful—I reach out and *grab* it. I'd been exposed to enough hospital procedures that the sight of surgical masks and IV tubes didn't scare me, and I liked the idea of attacking my renegade cancer aggressively. As I waited for the anesthesia to take hold in the OR, the last thing I remembered was a nurse asking, "No eating or drinking since midnight? No contact lenses, false teeth, spare parts or extras?" Once I was out, I'd be flipped onto my stomach so they could get to my hips, where the marrow is easily accessible and there's enough available to get in one sitting. But 99.9 percent of it is useless, because they're interested only in stem cells, which have the capacity to become everything else: red cells, white cells, and platelets. Stem cells are rare, and there's no real way to identify them. So they make several holes on each side of the pelvis and stick a needle in dozens of times until they get enough—the amount is proportionate to an individual's weight, but it's about a quart. It's filtered and collected in a bag, where it's mixed with a preservative and an anticoagulant so it doesn't form little dumplings.

I woke up quite sore but went back to work that afternoon. The few people who knew I'd just been drilled with seven holes under general anesthesia looked like they were seeing a ghost. Maybe I didn't want to capitulate to any pain or fatigue then because of some foreboding that the tougher stuff was still ahead. And I had to prepare the staff for the time I'd be away. August is traditionally a low-key month, and most of the sittings had been piggybacked onto earlier assignments in anticipation of vacation schedules, so there would be no need to micro-manage. Most of my friends were away, sparing me endless explanations about my whereabouts, and my staff was so capable that I knew they could get on without me. But I wasn't planning to be very ill. I was quite expecting editorial meetings around my bed every day. Hah! Little did I know ...

Most of what is needed to replenish the blood comes from the marrow, but as a kind of backup the doctors wanted "peripheral cells" from the circulating blood. Red blood cells last about 120 days, and platelets last about a week, but white blood cells last only seven hours, so the peripheral cells are stored in case the bone marrow remaining in the body fails down the line when the white count has bottomed out. Back at the hospital and awake this time, I was hooked up to a machine that spun some blood out of my body with centrifugal force, isolating the stem cells and returning the rest, like factory seconds. All the talk about marrow made me think of osso buco, but actually I'd been mainlining cheese at the doctor's instruction to build up the calcium in my bones, and I chewed Tums all during this procedure for the same reason.

It seemed like a bad joke, but I was suddenly homeless again. The house we'd been renting from Mike Nichols was sold, and our new rental wouldn't be vacated and painted for several months, so all of our possessions were once again packed into cartons for storage. My heart was breaking as I watched the men in my life head for the beach while I set up migrant camp in the Carlyle Hotel, with a surrogate family in the form of room service (who probably thought I was feeding a pet mouse from all the cheese plates I ordered). It can be rather chic to live in a hotel, like Eloise at the Plaza, but it offers no semblance of home. I'd think of a favorite book or bracelet or T-shirt and realize that it was packed away in the bowels of the storage company. Friends were making plans for Martha's Vineyard, and I was planning for Mount Sinai. I got a piano in my suite and calmed myself with Clementi and Sibelius, with Scott Joplin rags and Christmas carols from a Methodist hymnbook. (Anyone who over heard must have thought: *Christmas in July?*) But the reason piano playing is so therapeutic is that while you're doing it, you can't think of anything else.

For one night that July, I slept at the White House. After working with Hillary Rodham Clinton on Kids 4 Kids, I knew that I wanted to do an article in *Bazaar* about her thoughts on children, marriage, health, and other subjects that politicians often refer to in a dismissive way as "women's issues." She agreed to talk if I would conduct the interview myself, and extended an invitation to stay the night in the Lincoln Bedroom. A presidential car picked me up at National Airport, drove up the circular drive at 1600 Pennsylvania Avenue, and deposited me right at the South Portico of the White House, the site I had seen in so many newsreels, where so many famous feet had crossed the portal. A special assistant to the president took me upstairs to my room, dominated by Abraham Lincoln's huge mahogany bed covered with a gold spread, and a facsimile copy of the Gettysburg Address on the desk. My sitting room was the place where Richard Nixon wrote his resignation speech in front of one of his famous fires. Not one of our most energy-efficient leaders, he preferred to turn the air conditioning on high and keep the fires lit in summer.

First I called everyone I know—my husband, children, mother, office, the butcher, the baker, the lady who sold me Milk Flake bars when I was a child—to squeal, "Guess where I am?" Then I wandered the house and grounds. As a guest of the first lady, I had a badge that permitted access to any part of the building and grounds except the Clintons' personal living quarters. I saw the dogwood tree planted in honor of the Oklahoma City bombing victims and the magnolia tree into which a renegade plane had once crashed. Everywhere I went, the Secret Service men would follow me, whispering into walkie-talkies: "Guest leaving Rose Garden and entering South Lawn . . ."

Later that afternoon, my interview with the first lady was held in the beautiful yellow Oval Room decorated by Jackie Kennedy. Mrs. Clinton was writing what would become her best-selling book *It Takes a Village* and talked about the welfare of women and children worldwide, about mentors and health care and female management styles, and about a radical bank in Bangladesh that had started making loans to poverty-level people without any

227

collateral, only to discover that women are better credit risks. It was a wide-ranging conversation, and a wonderful interview. I brought the tapes back and edited out my painful ahhs and umms; her long replies were perfect. Toward the end of the interview I had gotten very brave. Knowing the problems Mrs. Thatcher had had with the British press's comments in regard to her hair and clothing, I decided to ask Mrs. Clinton about her hairstyles. Hillary Rodham Clinton has fun with her hair. Nothing anyone has said or written has made her stop changing it. In fact, she was trying another style then, in the summer of 1995. Here is what she told me on the subject:

"Now this, as my husband says, is one of his favorite hairstyles, because it is what I wore in high school. I didn't know him in high school, but he has my graduation picture. It's always been one of his favorite pictures, and the other day he said, 'Oh, this is wonderful—you're back to your high school hair.'

"Hair to me has always been the one part of my body that I had control over. I could not grow any taller, I could not lengthen my legs, I could not make my eyes have perfect vision—there was nothing else I could really do. But my hair has always been a source of great amusement to me. I've cut it, permed it, highlighted it, worn it short, worn it long. I was always having fun with it, and I never realized it would be such a serious subject. I mean, do you wear the same clothes every year? Even if you think you've got your style down pat, you still want some slight variation. Accessorize it, do something with it—well, that's the way I feel about my hair." Ironically, she was talking to a woman about to enter a bone marrow transplant and lose every strand of hair on her body.

At dinner that night with Lisa Caputo, the first lady's press secretary, and Ann Stock, her social secretary, I was warned that the Clintons might knock at my door to say good night, so I kept my makeup on, but I had no midnight visitors, just red-rimmed eyes the next morning. Out the window of the Lincoln Bedroom, I saw the president go jogging with a group of students, but I relaxed with my breakfast, ordered the night before, of poached eggs on toast and All-Bran. That I was one of the few Britons to sleep in the Lincoln Bedroom posed an irony that did not escape Mrs. Clinton, who commented that the last time my compatriots were at the White House, they burned the place down. I apologized profusely.

Finally, on July 26, there was a vacancy in the BMT unit. It was already a full day on my calendar. I had agreed to be photographed that morning for a *New York* magazine story on the fashion press, and I saw no reason to cancel. With all the attention to my hair and makeup, I thought at least there'd be one decent picture of me if I died. We'd scheduled a staff picnic in my office to celebrate the on-schedule completion of our fat September issue themed around women in the year 2000. That afternoon I was called to a meeting of Hearst executives, where momentous changes in the company were announced.

Magazines guarantee their advertisers a certain level of readership, an estimated number of eyeballs every month, and charge for advertising according to those numbers. In an effort to offset unprecedented increases in paper and postal costs, Hearst decided to print fewer copies and raise ad rates and newsstand prices for most of its magazines, hoping to eliminate what were termed "marginal readers": those who bought subscriptions below cost and thus were deemed expendable to advertisers. Readers who are committed to paying full price, it was argued, are more brand-loyal and have more disposable income. The move was described as "dramatic," "sweeping," and "bold" by the *Wall Street Journal* but provoked criticism from the advertising community, where the response was: Who the hell do you think you are? *Bazaar* was less affected than those magazines that depended on advertising from mass companies such as Kraft Foods, which immediately instructed its agencies to take its business elsewhere. In hindsight, I believe this reconfiguration was launched naively. It should have been done quietly and independently by each magazine, nurturing the advertisers and explaining the new policy to them. Instead, the news was put out as a big press release, and the damage control continued for two years.

To hear about such serious corporate number-crunching, I was wearing a serious suit and heels that added several inches to my stature. But Calvin Klein and Prada seemed a bit excessive for the hospital, so after the meeting, I changed into my J. Crew sweats and J. P. Tod's moccasins to check in to the isolation ward of the BMT unit at Mount Sinai, with Andrew by my side. The room was plain and gray, with a distant view of the Cathedral of St. John the Divine across Central Park. Since this would be home for a while, I'd been told to bring my favorite creature comforts. I actually packed exercise weights, thinking I'd do curls in my spare time (Hah! and Hah!), plus a navy-and-white Ralph Lauren comforter. But no family photos. I never travel with them because they make me cry.

I started chemo the next day, Andrew's birthday. Almost immediately I couldn't eat anything, but I looked bloated from the IV feedings, which provide plenty of fluid to flush the drugs out of one's system. I expected to become bald, but did not anticipate my neck swelling like a sumo wrestler's and my lips puffing out like a Ubangi warrior's. Chemotherapy, I was told, destroys rapidly changing cells, which is considered to be the essence of cancer, but these same rapidly changing cells are also what make up hair and skin and the lining of the mouth and stomach. My mouth became ulcerated and I couldn't swallow my own saliva, so I was given a small device to vacuum out my mouth. I knew I was dribbling, but I didn't care. My pale skin turned scarlet. Every day brought some new horrifying change to my body. But the worst of it was the shaking chills. That was an antibody response called "rigor"— a reaction to the donor platelets I was given while waiting for my body to make its own. At any one time there were three bags of stuff going into me, and my system revolted. It started with uncontrollable shivers, which got bigger and bigger, like an epileptic seizure. If I had visitors, I had to say, "You'd better leave." Having seen the reaction on my husband's face when it happened, I didn't want to frighten anyone else.

I couldn't have flowers—in isolation, everything in the room had to be sterile—so people sent books, music, and films on tape, most of which sat ignored and unused. I kept trying to snap into alertness, but part of the affront of this treatment was losing my cognitive self, as well as my physical self. Dozing was easy, but sleeping was not. The pain medication was so wildly hallucinogenic that I was in my own private Woodstock, joined perhaps by the patient in the next room, who called to inform me that the nurses were having a hashish party. Andrew says that I reported having phantom visitors, or he'd find me wandering around half-naked, the blinds wide open, making plangent noises to nobody in particular. Grace Coddington came to visit often, but one day I gave her new, elaborate, and totally fictional directions to my room, sending her roaming through the labyrinthine corridors of the hospital for an hour. At one point I was sobbing uncontrollably because I was convinced that I was to be the guest of honor at a charity benefit going on in the hall, but nobody came to get me in my wheelchair. I kept asking, "How was the party?"

I don't even remember how loony I was, but apparently it got pretty bizarre. I'd call the office and say, "They're killing me," or launch into reveries about my childhood, or talk about five different things at the same time. My friends were valorous: Since anyone who visited had to be covered from head to toe with mask and gown, I couldn't tell what they were wearing, but Annemarie Iverson would get a pedicure (beauty editors know where to get the best ones) and wear sandals so I could peek at her toes and talk about shoes. Even when I couldn't talk, I loved hearing gossip from work, about how X's pregnancy was going or what misbegotten outfit Y was wearing or why Z had come in with a hangover. Paul Cavaco, then a fashion director, would call to entertain me with style news, interspersed with exquisitely detailed narratives about oral sex. *Every* conversation with Paul ended up being about sex. We'd be talking about high heels, which led to "fuck-me shoes," and suddenly it became an anything-but-sketchy description of who was doing what to whom, and whether it was good or bad. Unfortunately, I wasn't taking notes. Of course, my exercise weights sat in the closet—I couldn't even wash what remained of my hair—but I did have occasional bursts of strength. Once I asked Annemarie to bring batteries for a radio. She couldn't

231

get them out of the package with rubber gloves on her hands so I grabbed a pair of medical scissors and ripped them open.

I stopped looking in the mirror because I no longer recognized the face or body I saw. I'd always had a little mole on my breast, and I watched it turn coal black. Very Cindy Crawford of me, but I realized I was being fried from the inside out. I was reduced to an almost animal level of survival, struggling just to make it through the day, all privacy and dignity gone, trying to hold on to something that represented the routine of life I'd taken for granted. Once I asked for a cup of tea (made with sterilized water), but I didn't have the strength to hold it, and the scalding water spilled on my stomach. I had burned, blistering skin for weeks and still bear the scars. Everything I ate or drank spilled on my nighties. I hated the hospital gowns—it felt like the ultimate humiliation to be wearing that ugly, flimsy garb—so Andrew ran a laundry service, bringing me cleaned and pressed Brooks Brothers nightshirts. My worst nightmare was having to wear something soiled, so I tried washing them in the tiny bathroom sink, but it was too exhausting, and a nurse had to finish for me. I got to hate the sight of the nurses, arriving almost hourly with little beakers of fluid to make the medicine go down. The pills got bigger, and I got angrier and threw them away. The only time I laughed was when a large black nurse saw my silver-blond wig sitting in the corner and put it on. But as soon as Andrew walked in the door, I'd begin to weep.

Andrew spent most of his time on the Long Island Express—way, traveling back and forth between me and the boys. I'd been encouraged to have my children visit, the reasoning being that there's already a degree of upheaval in a family from the cancer diagnosis, and kids can have disturbing fantasies about what's going on. Social workers feel that there should be some exposure, that kids do better knowing what they're dealing with, but I felt I looked too disfigured, like a Hieronymus Bosch painting of someone seen by the light of the flames of hell. Andrew felt the boys wouldn't want to see me like that. *He* didn't want to see me like that. The hospital even offered us the use of a videophone: one set up in my room, one at home, so we could visit face to face, but Andrew pretended he couldn't get it to work. The boys stayed at camp, distracted as much as possible by sailing and tennis, sending me handmade cards and notes with pictures of themselves. Only short calls were possible, a few brief reassurances of love escaping my swollen and deformed mouth. Andrew fielded their constant questions, lying, of course, and playing down the gravity of my condition, putting on weight himself from stress.

Some of my friends later confessed that they were furious with Andrew for not spending more time at the hospital, but I wouldn't have wanted him hovering, attempting to conceal his horror and dismay in an imperfect pretense of equanimity. I know it may sound heartless to any woman who, in similar circumstances, would want her husband at fixed coordinates beside the hospital bed, but that's not the sort of deal Andrew and I have. If he'd put a cot in the room, I would have thought I wasn't expected to wake up. He was trying in his own way to make me feel things were normal. I did *sometimes* feel ignored. He'd say, "I'm going out to hear some jazz tonight, so don't call me too early in the morning." Of course he was too worried about me to go, but I'd call the next day crying, "You don't love me anymore." I thought it was mean that he would come and go so quickly, not realizing that I had dozed off in the interim and that this visit was his sixth of the day! I remembered reading that Newt Gingrich had left his first wife when she was having chemotherapy. That possibility is in the back of your mind at such a black time. You feel you're never going to bake another pie, never going to help your kids with their homework, never going to walk down a beach, never going to make love again. You think: What kind of a terrible mother/wife/boss am I, not supporting anyone, being so needy and helpless?

What Andrew did was shield me as much as possible from the feeling of being institutionalized, bringing from the video store the "mushy" movies I'm usually forbidden to rent. He offered miso soup, hoping that my love of Japanese food would stoke my appetite, and canned mandarin oranges, hoping that the vitamin C would have a palliative effect on my system. But I couldn't eat any real food, not even the Jell-O that arrived with every tray (under

233

the *best* of circumstances, Jell-O is not a great palate teaser). Breakfast, lunch, and dinner came from a bag of green liquid pumped through an IV tube. (I don't even want to think about why it was green.) Mostly I sat by the window. I knew the exact time the sun rose and set, the glow from traffic lights and summer humidity. I couldn't see people on the street, only buildings, so the landscape looked like a scene from *The X-Files*. I thought: *This must be what it's like to be in prison.*

By mid-August, I was improving enough to be excited when I heard people out in the hallway donning surgical gloves, thinking: *Maybe they're coming to see me.* Lonely and bored and longing to get some work done, I had a fax machine installed in my room and storyboards of *Bazaar* layouts taped to the walls. It was a great treat to have my staff come for meetings, with everyone wearing masks and looking like aliens (we took ridiculous Polaroids), although *I* should have been masked so I didn't scare people. I could still barely talk because of the sores in my mouth, so I'd grunt, a gormless creature pretending I was making decisions. They probably went back to the office wondering, "What the *hell* was she saying?" One regrettable executive decision from that time haunts me still: a cover logo so bland and washed-out that we now refer to it as Pink Paleface. I was insistent—it was subtle, regal, I would not be talked out of it.

Finally I was out of isolation, but my platelet count was still low, a condition with the lovely name of thrombocytopenia, which means your blood won't clot and you can bleed uncontrollably. A normal count is 100,000; mine was 30,000, and I couldn't go home until it reached 75,000. One day the Princess of Wales called for a chat, and when the platelet count was done again in the afternoon, it was 80,000, and I was discharged. So I believe the princess was single-handedly responsible for getting me home, and no one will ever convince me otherwise.

The ordeal was over, or so I thought, in the last week of August. My skin was ash-gray and my tongue had green moss growing on it, but the doctors said I could go home, out to the beach for Labor Day. That was the weekend of a terrible fire that ravaged thousands of acres on Long Island, and what should have been a ninety-minute drive took four hours, a journey so enervating that I could barely make the walk across the room to greet Robbie and Chris that I'd been practicing. I'd been so afraid that I'd see horror or revulsion in their faces, but I needn't have feared. Our reunion was joyous—no tears, just hoots and whoops and hugs—but I had to hug them from around the back to avoid germs. I wasn't strong enough for any sort of celebration. Simply hearing their voices or their favorite TV programs made me happy.

Leaning on Andrew, I'd go down to the narrow strip of beach at the back of our house each morning and sit on my favorite rock with a cup of tea, often so weak that he'd have to carry me back. In what was a real family tragedy, Sophie, one of our Labradors, had recently died—she actually suffocated when she stuck her nose in a big bag of dog food she pulled out of the trash—and the other dog, Samantha, had become quite attached to me, and her loyalty redoubled when she perceived how weak I was. Andrew would try taking her for a run on the beach, but even after he dragged her on a leash, she'd break away and run back to me. (It was while he was running with the dog's leash wrapped around his arm that he got the idea for a unique exercise device that he has now patented and is in the process of trying to manufacture as "Ten-Tor," which has helped him to lose forty pounds without dieting and has got him "in the best shape of my life.")

It was a warm Labor Day weekend, but I was sitting outside on the patio with Grace Coddington. I was freezing cold and starting to feel my body burning from the inside out. Andrew took my temperature every five minutes and called Peter Dottino when it hit 100 degrees. He managed to rouse a kindly Long Island pharmacist for an after-hours prescription, but the medicine didn't work, and I had to return to the hospital. Andrew called a car service so he could tend to me in the backseat, and I sobbed hysterically the whole way into the city, repeating over and over, "Why am I so sick? Why am I so sick?" It turned out that I had an infection under the skin where the Broviac had been placed to administer the chemo during my BMT. Although it was a relatively minor setback, it was one of my lowest points. During that whole long month in isolation, I'd told myself I could endure anything with a finite horizon to it, an end in sight, but I hadn't figured on a relapse, and I didn't have any leftover pluck or fortitude to deal with it. It was the only time during the whole Grand Guignol experience that I would cry into my pillow for hours on end, wretched and inconsolable, wondering how I could last another day. Watching Andrew leave my hospital room brought back memories of saying goodbye to my parents at boarding school, watching them walk away and thinking for a brief moment that I might never see them again. And, although this sounds like too much of a soap opera to mention, it was my birthday. Andrew had been too anxious to think about it, and no one remembered either. There were no presents, no cake, no cheer.

The day I finally went home was moving day for the whole family, into our new brownstone. The scene was chaotic—cartons piled up to the ceiling, windows taken out to get an armoire in. Most of the packing had gone on without me, and I was so weak, I couldn't lift a finger to help with the unpacking. I had to trust to Andrew's and the boys' instincts about where things should go— to this day I still haven't figured out where some of my favorite pots and pans are living. All of my summer clothes had been left in storage at the beach, but it was still hot in New York, so I lay on the bed in T-shirts purloined from other people's drawers. I'd lost much more weight, forty-five pounds since the original diagnosis of cancer, and I hadn't even begun to build back my strength.

What can I say about the irony of the "Cancer Diet"? For twenty years I knew that I was fat, but I never realized there was a thinner me inside. I'd tried working out at a gym, but I'd be in the locker room in my underwear, and somebody would ask me to look at her résumé. Mornings were too frenetic for a Jane Fonda video or a Nordic Track, and I dissolved at the end of a day—all typical excuses for sloth. My heart goes out to people who struggle with their weight as I did, because the world can be cruel. Magazines like *Bazaar* are accused of contributing to the problem, but we are in the business of presenting fashion, and we can't get around the fact that, with rare exception, clothes look best on a slim silhouette.

Cancer accomplished something that Weight Watchers never could, and I do love the fact that I don't have an extraneous bump anywhere. But I had to learn how to live in this new body, one with different tastes and different energy. The length of my digestive tract was "denuded" by chemo, from my mouth, where the food went in, to my ... well, you know where the food comes out. I couldn't eat anything that might have bacteria. No eggs, no shrimp, no salads or fruit washed by anybody else, nothing raw, nothing that was cooked yesterday, and no alcohol: Chemotherapy has the same effect on the liver as a Lost Weekend. For a while, carbonated water was too strong, and baby food was not bland enough. I was never hungry, but I was panicked about finding something to feed myself—a rather incongruous situation for someone who'd spent too many years denying herself food or feeling guilty about indulging. I lived on chicken noodle soup and cans of those "nutrition supplements" marketed to the elderly. My first restaurant meal, at Petrossian, was a scientific experiment: testing the restorative powers of caviar. I considered it a variation of tea and toast—with a little black jam on top—but my doctors were horrified: caviar is, of course, raw eggs. Anytime we went out, Andrew had to make sure nobody in the restaurant was sneezing or coughing, and he scoped out the exits like the Secret Service in case I started to choke and had to make a quick getaway.

I experienced a series of "firsts" that would seem innocuous to a healthy person but felt momentous to me, like being born again: the first time I had enough hair to shave my legs or use mascara, the first time I stood in line again for a movie, the first sushi, the first plane ride. Some funny things transpired: BMT destroyed my taste buds but gave me a soprano's vocal cords: Suddenly I could hit the top notes in "The Star-Spangled Banner," although the Yankees never called to request my services. My nails had stopped growing and fell out gradually during the treatment, and the growing-back process was excruciating—the pain would wake me in the middle of the night, and made it hard to get dressed. So Andrew had to help me pull my pantyhose on, which may be the most touching chore he's ever performed for me—he developed a definite technique. My hair started growing back, and he convinced me that I wasn't too old for the Jean Seberg look. But he's still waiting for me to gain weight. With a lascivious smile, he'll grab whatever handful of flesh he can find and tell me, "No man in his right mind fancies skinny women."

AS I WAS reminded by all those consent forms I signed, BMT is still a giant crapshoot, hopeful but essentially unproven until enough people have had the treatment to provide meaningful results. The National Cancer Institute has initiated a large-scale study of BMT in the treatment of breast cancer, but the data won't be known until the year 2000, and the ovarian cancer study didn't begin until January 1997: 275 women across the country who have some disease left at second-look surgery are being given BMT, according to a regime developed by Dr. Patrick Stiff, at Loyola University in Maywood, Illinois. Dr. Stiff insists that the gruesome toxic reaction I experienced is unusual, that most of his patients are back to regular routines of work and play in about three weeks. But one of the saddest things he sees is the number of women who go through this alone. Ovarian cancer is more likely to affect women who don't have children, and in many cases they're miles away from any family. It would have been unimaginable for me to embark on such a course without my family. Andrew was my right arm, my left foot, compensating for my reluctance or incapacity to absorb information. When I'd say, "I don't want to know," he'd want to know everything. And the boys gave me every reason to get better.

The innuendo surrounding my bone marrow transplant did not escape me. It was reported that ambitious editors nonchalantly sent their CVs to Hearst, and possible successors were mentioned in gossip mills, although Claeys Bahrenburg remained solidly behind me, never even appointing a deputy editor during my absence.

Teetering on the brink of death in order to save my life was a bittersweet odyssey. I heard from the team at Mount Sinai that BMT is often a transforming experience—not one that anyone would ever choose, but one that slyly becomes an impetus for growth. Some people make the decision to leave jobs or relationships that are emotionally toxic, and a lot of things get said in families that wouldn't otherwise be articulated. I've not done anything differently—that would feel like conceding to the cancer. I thrive on stress. I have a beloved but insane job, with its politics, its pressures, its egos and its attitudes, the tumult about which model or photographer gets to fly Concorde, the hissy fits about which writer's words are edited, the personnel changes. There have been ripples and shocks: In 1996, Paul Cavaco, one of my fashion directors, called me from a sitting to say he was going to *Vogue*. I didn't mind the message so much as the method of delivery—isn't it decreed by etiquette authorities that you don't break up with someone on the phone? And I had already got a new boss myself: In January 1996, Cathie Black, the dynamic former president and CEO of the Newspaper Association of America, took over Hearst magazines, replacing Claeys Bahrenburg, who is now the vice-chairman of Petersen Publishing. When I'm not working, I lie awake in the middle of the night worrying about my children, my magazine, my planet. I don't know that I could lower the stress level. I don't know that I want to lower the stress level.

But I'm also very good at time out, and I take much joy in my life, a quantity that is universally acknowledged to be an instrument of healing. At the end of a crazy day, I retreat to the anodyne activities of family life: making farmhouse stew with dumplings while sipping a glass of white wine over ice, helping Chris with his vocabulary test and talking to Robbie about Rollerblading, watching *NYPD Blue* or *Seinfeld* with Andrew and falling asleep during the news. It's mundane, it's boring, it's heaven. It's my real life with my family—a peaceful, sacrosanct time, with candles on the mantel and flowers on the table and linen, never paper, napkins. And we *never* discuss fashion or magazines. Outside of this escape hatch, I live in a mad, mad, mad, mad world, and I love it. But I won't put up with nonsense anymore, even from myself: There is no such thing as a bad hair day for me. Most of us walk around feeling immortal, which is normal and important. But I've seen the dark side of the moon and will never take the fact of life for granted.

# 15

PEOPLE SOMETIMES ASK Andrew whether it was difficult for him when I decided to go public about cancer, and he always answers, "*We* decided." We had a consensus about sacrificing some of our privacy if it might spare other women and their families our pain and trauma, even help to save lives. I'm a journalist—I believe that information is power. But I recognize the fine line between giving people information and terrifying them.

The news about a possible link between ovarian cancer and fertility drugs has scared the hell out of people: the women who have taken these drugs or are contemplating it, and the doctors treating them. Fertility specialists often speak in glowing terms about the rewards of their branch of medicine, helping couples achieve a dream through the miracle of science. But we also live in a litigious society, and doctors whose practices were being called into question in newspaper headlines were worried about covering their asses. When the first study implicating the use of fertility drugs in the development of ovarian cancer was published in the medical literature, the initial response from the American Society for Reproductive Medicine read like a circling of wagons around the camp: A memo from the president to the member doctors mentioned "concern" but concluded that the study was "flawed." One of the leading British fertility experts said, "The Whittemore paper is widely recognized as an extremely poor study. There is very little reason to suppose there is a link."

Infertility is big business these days. According to the ASRM, 1.3 million American women are treated each year, and the fees they pay are high. Depending on what part of the country you're in, an initial visit with a fertility specialist runs several hundred dollars. Add thousands more for diagnostic tests, blood work, ultrasounds, possibly a hysterosalpingogram (dye is injected into the uterus through the cervix and X-rayed to see if it flows out the fallopian tubes, proving they're not blocked). Clomiphene citrate (of which Clomid is one brand) costs about $30 for five days each cycle. Pergonal costs about $50 per injectable ampule, and you may use one or two a day for seven to twelve days, even more. If the drugs actually work and you produce viable eggs, the cost skyrockets. A 1994 study published in the *New England Journal of Medicine* reported that the average cost of a single in vitro fertilization is $8,000, and the price is not going down.

The odds are fair to poor that these costly potions will work. The rate of pregnancy resulting in a live birth in 1993 was 18.3 percent for each IVF procedure. The rate is much lower, probably around 5 percent, for women over forty, a constituency that represents avid, often desperate, customers of reproductive technology. There is no single accepted national standard for computing the rate of success. Fertility clinics and programs are profit-making enterprises, often involved in competitive self-promotion, sometimes advertising, and they can do creative math. But a pregnancy and a baby are not the same thing. Some programs define pregnancy as a positive urine test, and a chemical pregnancy like the one I had once is not uncommon after IVF. And some clinics enhance their take-home-baby rates by counting twins (also fairly common) as two successful pregnancies, not one.

Fertility treatment is an unregulated industry that seems to operate according to its own rules. There is no governing body setting standards of treatment or establishing what constitutes informed consent about a perceived risk of cancer, no thread of commonality for doses of drugs, duration, intervals, anything. What is done in New York may be vastly different from what is done in London or anyplace else—that's why interpreting statistics is so difficult. The package inserts for Clomid and Serophene, the two major brands of clomiphene citrate, warn against use for more than three cycles, the guidelines under which the manufacturers got FDA approval. If the drug works, your probability of getting pregnant is the same as for the normal population, and 50 percent of couples trying to conceive the old-fashioned way will be pregnant within three months of trying. If you don't respond in that time, more workup is indicated, not more drugs. The practice guidelines from the American Society for Reproductive Medicine (ASRM) for its member physicians suggest a limit of six cycles before further evaluation, continuing to six more cycles if all the studies are normal. The package insert for Pergonal recommends no more than five courses of treatment. I had nine cycles of that drug, which is not unusual even today. A recent book by a fertility expert admits that the older the woman, the more Pergonal will be required to stimulate the development of follicles—if she's over forty, it's almost always "necessary" to use from four to ten ampules a day, way over the manufacturer's recommendation. Dr. Benjamin Younger, the executive director of the ASRM, admits that probably half of all drug prescriptions in this country are off-label: Doctors increase the dose for patients and treat them for longer than is recommended.

The FDA now requires manufacturers to include these words of caution: "Prolonged use of clomiphene may increase the risk of a borderline or invasive ovarian tumor." Pergonal includes no such warning, since it was not implicated in the early studies about fertility drugs and cancer. Its packaging includes this diluted message: "There have been infrequent reports of ovarian neoplasms, both benign and malignant, in women who have undergone multiple drug regimens for ovulation induction; however, a causal relationship has not been established." Not yet. In theory, the implications are even greater: A woman taking clomiphene is unlikely to produce more than three eggs in one month, but with Pergonal it can be many more, and it is the rupturing of that many follicles that is a potential problem.

In 1993, after that first shocking study became public knowledge, three researchers from the National Institute of Child Health and Human Development wrote an article in the *ASRM Journal*. "At present," they said, "there is no need to change medical practice regarding the use of fertility-enhancing drugs. There is enough cause for concern, however, to slightly alter the physician's approach to counseling patients. We suggest advising patients receiving fertility drugs as to the possible increased risk of ovarian cancer."

No such advisory exists in Great Britain, where the Human Fertilisation & Embryology Authority (HFEA), the government body that licenses fertility clinics, issues a code of practice, as well as a patient's guide. The code, which is reviewed and revised about every eighteen months, states that clients should have information about "the possible side effects and risks of the treatment to the woman and any resulting child," and the patient's guideline (1996 edition) states that prospective patients should be given written information "about any risks involved," but neither document mentions ovarian cancer, leaving it up to the discretion of individual practitioners to determine what constitutes informed consent. My former fertility specialist, Professor Ian Craft, offers a glossy twenty-four-page booklet about his clinic, the London Gynaecology & Fertility Centre, which mentions the possible complications of anesthesia, miscarriage, ectopic pregnancy, multiple pregnancy, and ovarian hyperstimulation (where the ovaries enlarge and develop fluid-filled cysts). But the subject of ovarian cancer is not raised, and the drugs used to induce ovulation for IVF are said to have "very few side effects." There is nothing "categorical" in the research, no "proof positive" about the risk of cancer, according to Craft. "With short-term clomiphene, I don't think there is an increased risk," he says, "but with long-term, there probably is, if the reports are correct. It may be true of Pergonal too, but I don't know about it. The fact is, we're not having any directives from the HFEA."

I can't accept this argument, and I don't think we can afford to wait. I realize that doctors prefer hypotheses to be carved in granite before adapting them to clinical practice, but I fear we are writing them in the blood of women whose lives will be sacrificed to the due process of scientific investigation. "There is prima facie evidence that ovarian stimulation causes ovarian cancer," says Dr. Ian Jacobs, director of the Gynaecological Cancer Research Unit at St. Bartholomew's and the Royal London Hospitals, who in April 1997 led the first international conference on ovarian cancer detection. "I don't think the question is answered, but it's biologically plausible, it makes sense, and what data there are suggest that it's a real effect. I think we actually have a responsibility to be proactive. Feeling bad, like we have been up until this very minute, isn't really adequate. Women should be making sure they are informed, and we should be banging on the doors of the HFEA, insisting that they are. Not that women shouldn't have ovarian stimulation, but they should be given the information that there may be a risk."

I think there should be some door-banging in the United States too. The current ASRM "guidelines for the provision of infertility services," which are reviewed and revised every few years, remind physicians considering the value of treatment that "the adverse effects could be serious" and that "the right choice for a given couple" will depend, among other considerations, on "their approach to risk-taking." There is no standardized consent form or language of disclosure. A patient guide published by the ASRM in 1995 now includes this paragraph:

A recent study suggested that women who use ovulation drugs such as clomiphene citrate and HMG may be at increased risk for ovarian cancer. It is not currently known if a risk exists, but this study shows that more research is needed to determine if there is a causal relationship between the use of ovulation drugs and ovarian cancer. If a risk does exist, it is not known whether the risk is due to being infertile and anovulatory or to not conceiving, or if the risk is limited to a certain class of drugs, to a certain duration of use, or to the amount of use. This ill-defined suggested risk must be weighed against the risk of not being treated and not conceiving. Pregnancy and childbirth have always been associated with clear-cut medical risks, but most women willingly assume these risks because of their desire to have a child. Patients should discuss this topic with their physician in order to get an up-to-date perspective.

Put on such notice, I don't know how most women would react, if a "most women" reaction even exists. How many women longing for a baby would forgo treatment because of potential extra risk ten or twenty years down the pike? When I was taking fertility drugs, I doubt that such a vague caveat could have dissuaded me. That's fair—people make personal and arbitrary decisions about risk and benefit all the time in their lives. You recognize the risks associated with smoking, or sunbathing, or skydiving, and you decide how important the activity is, what you'll get out of it, what margin of safety makes you comfortable. Perhaps you go into denial mode to override apprehension or common sense. "Fear of ovarian cancer is not something patients process at a high level," says Dr. Younger of the ASRM. "The desire to reproduce is strong, and that makes them ripe for exploitation."

It's one thing for a woman to risk her health pursuing her desire to be a mother. But what about egg donors—those usually young and healthy women who, for whatever financial remuneration or personal satisfaction, undergo repeated cycles of fertility drugs to stimulate hyperovulation? The idea of sperm donation, for a couple whose infertility problem rests with the male partner, has been around for several hundred years and involves no risk to the donor—we all know exactly what it involves—although now the sperm can be frozen and preserved for later use. But the fertility drugs used in egg donation involve the same risk to the donor as they do to an infertile woman taking them. The paper from the National Institute of Child Health and Human Development extends

246

concern to these women: "Especially careful consideration should be given to counseling women who wish to donate eggs, particularly repeat donors, because they derive no reproductive benefit from their fertility drugs exposure."

My own oncologist, Peter Dottino, reminds me that the scientific data still do not support my deeply held belief that my cancer was linked to blasting my ovaries with fertility drugs, but he acknowledges that the infertility community initially reacted to that possibility the same way the U.S. government first responded to Gulf War Syndrome: Deny, deny, deny. "It was stupid," he says. "Even though they may ultimately admit there's a problem, the ill will and mistrust engendered by that kind of behavior takes generations to overcome." A researcher in Pennsylvania told me that she wrote to a local hospital suggesting that it call in all the women who had been treated for infertility there and screen them for ovarian cancer, using the CA-125 blood test and transvaginal ultrasound, the two most useful, albeit limited, means of detection. She presented the idea that this would be wonderful for public relations, demonstrating the hospital's ongoing concern for patients, and it would help her research as well. She never got an answer. The general feeling was that the hospital didn't even want to raise the questions.

It's reasonable to ask why these questions weren't raised *before* the horse left the barn. When new drugs come out, of course, they have gone through FDA review for possible harmful effects, but typically cancer isn't one of the harmful effects that the FDA tries to ensure against. "That's because it tends to be such a long-term complication," explains Dr. Mary Anne Rossing. "They couldn't have done the research linking fertility drugs with ovarian cancer, at least in humans, until the drugs were on the market for a while. They do look at data on animal testing, but it would be awfully difficult to ever get a drug approved if what we wanted the FDA to do was sit and watch what happens to people, even if there were volunteers."

Since there has been a suspicion of risk since 1991, I believe women deserve that information. If, as a fully informed adult, you desire to have a child much more than you fear ovarian cancer in the future, you might at least want to consider stopping short of the twelve cycles of treatment that were identified with increased risk in the most recent study. Or you might decide to proceed more directly to adoption.

And if you feel you're at higher risk, I'd advise you to be vigilant for the rest of your life. Don't skip regular pelvic exams or ignore persistent symptoms: constant and progressive bloating, having to wear sweatsuits because nothing else fits, indigestion, sometimes back pain, getting full fast, getting up to pee often at night. Despite the common perception that ovarian cancer is "silent" until it's too late, several studies confirm that this is not the case. There are symptoms, albeit vague and elusive, common with even Stage I disease. I don't want to send women running for blood tests every time they burp or change dress size, but most women diagnosed with ovarian cancer report having felt vaguely bad for about six months, as I did. There's a visceral lousiness, but you can't focus on what it is. Talk to your doctor about it. And if your doctor blows you off, find another.

It's true that there are still more questions than answers for women who are considered high-risk, and with a dearth of options, some have their ovaries removed *before* cancer can develop. But even such a draconian solution, called a prophylactic oophorectomy, isn't foolproof. There are known cases, undisputed in the scientific literature, of women getting ovarian cancer *after* their apparently healthy ovaries were removed. Pathologists can look at a slide of cancerous tissue to tell the site of origin, and these were cancers of organs that weren't even there. There's an explanation, of course: The cancer developed in the peritoneum, or abdominal lining, surrounding the ovaries. Some experts think that ovarian cancer is really more a cancer of the peritoneum, which gets trapped inside the ovary.

Seven years ago Ceil Sinnex of Paauilo, Hawaii, had prophylactic surgery after losing her grandmother, aunt, and cousins to the disease. She then founded Ovarian Plus International, a quarterly newsletter devoted to information about detection, screening, risk reduction, and the politics of ovarian cancer—and prevention, if we can all ever figure out what it is," says Sinnex. She believes that public ignorance resulting from the lack of a campaign with clout have relegated the disease to a position of ignored stepchild in the scientific community. "Ovarian cancer is so lethal and so disgracefully neglected that it is a modern curse," she says. "There is no early detection test because no relatively serious funding commitment has ever been made to find one."

Sinnex got the attention of her congresswoman, Representative Patsy Mink of Hawaii, who introduced the Ovarian Cancer Research Act of 1991 and several subsequent bills calling for more money to be appropriated at the National Institutes of Health. The efforts of Mink and others in Congress managed to increase federal funding more than fivefold, to $41 million for 1997. In 1993 the National Cancer Institute launched the Prostate, Lung, Colorectal and Ovarian Cancer (PLCO) Screening Trial, in which 150,000 volunteers at ten medical centers across the country, half of them women, will be "randomized," or selected by chance, and followed for ten years to determine whether certain screening techniques reduce the chance of dying from these diseases. For the ovarian part of the trial, the women will be monitored with CA-125 and transvaginal sonography. Half the participants will undergo these procedures, and half will receive routine care from their doctors.

Still, the PLCO trial is not the comprehensive study that many of those concerned with ovarian cancer wanted—for one thing, only women over fifty-five are included—and there is something of a consensus that the inclusion of ovarian cancer was an afterthought, that the inclusion of a female cancer was politically expedient for the NCI.

IN 1993 THE American College of Obstetrics and Gynecology stated that "to date, there are insufficient data to recommend any method of screening for ovarian cancer." In April 1994, the NIH Consensus Development Conference on Ovarian Cancer determined that most women do not need routine screening and risk unnecessary surgery if they insist out of fear on testing. Dr. Carmel Cohen of Mount Sinai says that is a shocking advisory and freely recommends transvaginal sonography screening to any woman who can afford it and who has access to skilled interpretation of the test (not a so-called "imaging center" along the lines of X-Rays-R-Us).

Respected, caring doctors still disagree about the value of the CA-125 test. It can be a Pandora's box, with unquelled anxiety ending in surgery. But Robert Bast, the doctor who developed the test, believes that this liability can be overcome with *repeated* tests. If you have a benign condition such as fibroids, your CA-125 might be up, but the next month it should go down. It certainly won't double. The pattern of benign conditions indicates that the numbers won't change progressively. Bast is working on a mathematical interpretation of test results so that doctors could take seriously a high CA-125 that was changing slowly or a low number that was changing rapidly. "I think we will soon identify a strategy that will detect early ovarian cancer," he says.

Such a strategy might include recommendations for a *baseline* CA-125, just as women are now encouraged to get a baseline mammogram so that doctors can track any changes in their breast tissue. Dr. Nicole Urban at the Fred Hutchinson Cancer Research Center in Seattle is trying to design a study that would show variations of CA-125 over time for an individual. Some women may hover around a low number, and some women may have a lot of fluctuation, but if you had a baseline CA-125 at age fifty or whenever you go through menopause, and then again a year later, the way the number has changed or not might be meaningful. Urban also has a proposal pending at the National Cancer Institute to address the anxiety about the imperfect capabilities of CA-125 testing: If women are screened for ovarian cancer, how will it affect their quality of life? Just because the test is imperfect, should it be dismissed as too stressful?

In April 1997, Ian Jacobs initiated a study of 120,000 healthy women throughout the United Kingdom to see whether screening

saves lives. Half the women will be screened, the others just followed, and the study will utilize a more sophisticated way of
looking at CA-125 results called ROC (risk of ovarian cancer):
Jacobs, along with several researchers at Harvard Medical School,
developed an algorithm, or mathematical computation, that indicates risk according to the results of the first CA-125 and the way
that number changes over time. Part of the funding comes from
the Centicor company, which manufactures the CA-125 test and
obviously has a vested interest, but Jacobs says he has been able to
ensure autonomy and believes the study will show the test's value.
"We need to cut down on the false positives," says Jacobs. "But if
we operate on women who have a positive CA-125 *and* a positive
sonogram, we'll only end up operating on 0.3 percent of the
population. We think the screening will save lives. We need to
prove it."

Some researchers believe that the quest for early detection is
futile and wrongheaded, that our best hope lies with prevention.
"Basically I think that women in their reproductive years should
be trying bitterly to get pregnant or be on the Pill," says Dr.
Andrew Berchuck of Duke University, who is studying the effect
of ovulation on cellular change. Berchuck identifies himself as one
of Ian Jacobs's best friends but feels that screening may be a hopeless
sort of endeavor. "Ovarian cancer is a terrible disease to screen
for," he argues. "It's uncommon, it's deep in the body, and there's
no well-defined risk group. You're looking for a needle in a
haystack. Screening is costly, and the best data we have say it's not
practical: Even if a test is positive, most of the time it's not cancer."
Indeed, I myself often pass Berchuck's advice on to other women:
The best thing she can do to prevent ovarian cancer is to have a
big family or be on the Pill.

Berchuck has become something of an evangelist for the Pill,
and certainly his message has put ovarian cancer in a different light
than breast cancer. "There's no lifestyle intervention that we know
can significantly alter your risk of breast cancer," he says. "Breasts
are accessible and changes can be seen, so screening and early detection may be the way to go. If there *were* some lifestyle change that

would reduce breast cancer by fifty percent, people would be shouting it from skyscrapers. Well, we've got something like that for ovarian cancer and nobody's shouting about it. Why? *People who get breast cancer live to lobby, and people with ovarian cancer don't.*"

Dr. Malcolm C. Pike of the University of Southern California in Los Angeles was a pioneer in showing how oral contraceptives protect against ovarian cancer by suppressing ovulation. "The risk goes down forever . . . and not just while you're taking the Pill," he emphasizes. (The Pill does not offer the same protection against breast cancer because breast tissue reacts differently to the hormones in the Pill.)

It's fair to say that the door has now been opened to plenty of investigation about ovarian cancer and reproductive health. The National Cancer Institute is sponsoring a study of 10,000 women who were treated at fertility clinics in five cities from the 1960s to the 1980s, chosen because their doctors were pioneers in the field, prescribing fertility drugs for long periods of time and at high doses before they were mainstream. "The effects of Clomid are consistent with theories about what causes ovarian cancer," says Dr. Rebecca Troisi, one of the project directors. "These women have been highly exposed. If there is an effect, it will be easier to see."

At the University of California in San Francisco, Dr. Mary Croughan-Minihane began in 1997 a three-year project tracing some 75,000 women treated at fifteen fertility clinics in California between 1965 and 1995, hoping to determine whether infertile women who take fertility drugs are at more risk for ovarian cancer than other infertile women. In order to tease out the possible effects of the drugs from infertility itself, this study will focus on four different groups: infertile women who've been treated with drugs; infertile women who've not been treated with drugs; fertile women who've received drugs so that ovulation can be more accurately timed and controlled for the purpose of artificial insemination (single mothers or lesbians or those whose husbands have a fertility problem); and very fertile young women who are egg donors. "My personal feeling is that it will have less to do with the diagnosis or cause of infertility and more to do with a woman's response to drugs," says Croughan-Minihane. "A woman taking Pergonal is very likely to produce nine, twelve, fifteen, twenty eggs [in one cycle]. If she's supposed to be releasing one egg and now she's releasing twelve, she's done the equivalent of one year's worth of ovulation in one month." That may be too much of a gamble for a woman already at higher risk, according to Croughan-Minihane. "If I saw a woman whose mother had died of ovarian cancer," she says, "I would pretty seriously counsel her against fertility drugs."

Since baby boomers, the first generation exposed to the Pill, are just entering the age of highest risk for ovarian cancer, Dr. Roberta Ness at the University of Pittsburgh is tracking the contraceptive histories of 500 women with ovarian cancer compared to 1,000 healthy women. Since oral contraceptives are thought to be highly protective against ovarian cancer, Ness is particularly interested in the birth-control practices of women who are very fertile versus those who are not.

Early in 1997, money was directed to ovarian cancer research by an unlikely benefactor: the U.S. Department of Defense. It turns out that the DOD has relatively deep pockets: $100 million for breast cancer, $38 million for prostate cancer, but only $7.5 million dollars for ovarian cancer. "It's the new kid on the block," says Colonel Irene Rich, director of the Army Medical Research Program, whose office allocates the grants. But Colonel Rich is a nurse who used to supervise the gynecologic oncology ward of Walter Reed Hospital, and she knows firsthand how important it is to *prevent* a disease that is so difficult to treat. She has gathered a blue-ribbon panel to offer advice in the grant-review process, including ovarian cancer survivors and their families, so that women personally affected by the disease can play a part in directing the research dollars.

Research is being done abroad as well: The Institut National de la Santé et de la Recherche Médicale is studying the use of fertility drugs among nearly all 4,000 patients diagnosed with ovarian cancer in France during one year. And at the Weizmann Institute of Science in Israel, researchers have developed an experimental chemotherapy for ovarian cancer that decreases the toxicity (and the devastating side effects) of cisplatin with "immunotargeting": Antibodies guide the drug molecules right toward the malignant cells, circumventing healthy tissue.

DESPITE MY PERSONAL passions, there are reasonable arguments *against* the implication of fertility drugs in this disease. Some studies (the most recent from the University of Copenhagen and the Danish Cancer Society, published in June 1997) show no increase of ovarian cancer among women treated with fertility drugs. Understand that there are actually several types of ovarian cancer: The overwhelming majority (about 85 percent) are *epithelial carcinomas* that originate in the covering of the ovaries. Much rarer are *granulosa tumors* that develop in the fibrous tissues holding the ovaries in place, and *germ cell cancers*, from cells that give rise to the ovaries during fetal development. Clomid and Pergonal have been implicated because of their effect on FSH, the follicle-stimulating hormone. But FSH does not act on epithelial cells at all: It acts on granulosa cells. So how could Clomid be a possible factor in the vast majority of ovarian cancers? It's an indirect effect. Even though the epithelium doesn't have receptors for the drug, Clomid is ultimately going to produce the rupturing that may lead to mutated cells.

But Dr. Paulsen and some other medical mavericks question whether ovulation and infertility are actually the culprits that increase the risk of ovarian cancer. Infertility generally means you're not ovulating, so why would that place you at increased risk? If less ovulation confers protection, that means there should be a strong correlation with age of menopause, but premature menopause doesn't seem to protect against ovarian cancer. Both tubal ligation (tying the fallopian tubes) and simple hysterectomy (removing the uterus but not the ovaries) *do* protect against ovarian cancer, even though you're still ovulating. Paulsen hypothesizes that it is actually endometriosis and other kinds of pelvic inflammation that lead to ovarian cancer. (I, of course, had pelvic inflammation in my early

254

twenties, yet another possible risk factor for ovarian cancer.) Endometriosis, which occurs when the lining of the uterus starts growing outside its usual place, is thought to be due to retrograde menstruation, the backward flow of menstrual fluid through the fallopian tubes into the pelvis, picking up "debris" along the way. This detritus may overwhelm the body's immune system, which is supposed to attend to abnormal cells and bacteria. It bathes the ovaries, perhaps stimulating the kind of repeated insult to cells that can initiate malignant change.

The more I look at all this information, the more I recognize the dichotomy between medical doctors and research scientists, with patients sometimes getting caught in the gap. "Most medicine is practiced ahead of science," says Paulsen. "Doctors think of a physiologic principle that works and then apply it. This is good— it allows the practice of medicine at the edge of knowledge. If we waited for scientific proof, we'd never use anything but aspirin and penicillin, which we *know* work. Epidemiologists, on the other hand, think that as long as they follow their rules, stay unbiased and honest, they will arrive at truth. Doctors believe that whatever you find out doesn't have that kind of certainty."

BUT AT LEAST and at last, the hot white light of research is beginning to shine on ovarian cancer.

# 16

ANY STORY ABOUT cancer is a palimpsest, written over many times, with the remnants of earlier stories imperfectly erased. Some you may know. There is the story of the actress Cassandra Harris, wife of actor Pierce Brosnan, who died of ovarian cancer in 1991 at age thirty-nine, and actress Sandy Dennis, who died in 1992 at age fifty-four, and singer-songwriter Laura Nyro, who died in 1997 at forty-nine. There is the story of Marina Baiul, the mother of Olympic ice skater Oksana Baiul, who never saw her daughter win a gold medal because she died of ovarian cancer at age thirty-six. Other stories are less well known: There is the story of Marsha Rivkin, who died at age forty-nine of ovarian cancer that eluded even her husband, a prominent Seattle oncologist. Her story is a worst-case scenario of the cobbler's family going barefoot, a scenario that Dr. Saul Rivkin is determined will *not* be repeated with any of his five daughters. In 1993 the family established the Marsha Rivkin Ovarian Cancer Research Center in Seattle, whose purpose is to reduce the ovarian cancer death rate by increasing public awareness, screening high-risk women, and raising funds with a

"Summer Run" that hopes to some day match the high-profile "Race for the Cure" for breast cancer.

But there are also stories about survivors. There is the story of Congresswoman Rosa DeLauro of Connecticut, diagnosed with ovarian cancer at age forty-three after complaining for months about lack of energy and flulike symptoms. At the time, she was chief of staff to Senator Christopher Dodd of Connecticut, about to manage his reelection campaign, and she had never been in a hospital. "When I finally had an ultrasound," she remembers, "I heard one physician say, 'There's the mass.' I said, ' "There's the mass"? This is an outrage—you've been examining me for months.' " Also determined that other women should be spared this misery, DeLauro has served on congressional committees to increase appropriations for research in genetics and screening, and has worked with pharmaceutical companies developing new chemotherapy drugs.

There is the story of Cindy Melancon, a nurse from Amarillo, Texas, diagnosed with ovarian cancer at age forty-two, who started a newsletter called *Conversations* to support women like herself through shared information. There is the story of Pam Faerber, a businesswoman from East Zionsville, Indiana, diagnosed at age forty-four, who started Ovar'Coming Together, a group providing networking for ovarian cancer survivors and education for all women regarding early warning signs and risks. And there is the story of Gail Hayward of Boca Raton, Florida, a mother of four diagnosed with ovarian cancer at age forty-seven, who went on to create the National Ovarian Cancer Coalition, a nonprofit organization bound and determined that by the year 2000, there will not be a woman or a doctor in this country unenlightened about the early, vague symptoms of the disease—spreading the message through seminars, schools, medical offices, and Web sites.

I serve as president of the Ovarian Cancer Research Fund, which honors the memory of Ann Schreiber, an administrator for the Department of Health and Human Services in New York before she died of ovarian cancer at age fifty-seven in 1994. Founded by

Ann's husband, Sol, to support research and education about the disease, the fund underwrites grants, provides community programs, and in 1996 commissioned a videotape for broadcast on public television. For the video, I introduced the stories of five women who have been diagnosed with the disease. It required a certain sangfroid to include myself as a cancer survivor in this company because, though I didn't admit it on camera, my own story is a work in progress.

In February 1996, six months after my bone marrow transplant, my CA-125 began to rise. Despite the most aggressive possible treatment, the ordeal and insult of highest-dose chemotherapy, a trace of cancer had returned. I got this news from Peter Dottino while I was on vacation with my family in Florida, and I steeled myself against crying in front of the children, but in private with Andrew I collapsed. It wasn't possible, it wasn't true, it wasn't fair. With the bone marrow transplant I had endured the worst kind of assault, a frightening, torturous experiment, and it had all been in vain. I walked around with dark glasses all week to hide my red eyes, unable to look at my sons without reliving the deepest fears of the cancer diagnosis, the apprehension about leaving them. Terror turned to self-flagellation: I'd look at my body in the bathtub, the tracery of my scars muted under the water, and think: *Failure. Fool. Defective wife and worse mother.*

When we returned to New York, I had a CAT scan from crotch to breasts, which showed nothing. But since CA-125 is such an accurate marker of cancer activity for me (way up when I was diagnosed, rapidly back to normal after surgery, up then down again after BMT), Dottino decided I needed another hit of chemo: this time Taxol, a new drug derived from the bark of the Pacific yew tree, approved by the FDA in 1992 to treat recurrent ovarian cancer. It takes about 30,000 pounds of bark to produce one kilogram of the drug, which can be used to treat about 500 patients. That adds up to about three trees per patient. Since this process is so difficult, time-consuming, and expensive, the National Cancer Institute has entered into a cooperative research and development agreement with Bristol-Myers Squibb to produce a synthetic, marketable form of the drug. (A similar drug is under development by the French company Rhone-Poulenc.) Taxol is unlike other chemotherapy drugs in that it paralyzes rather than destroys cancer cells, stabilizing the fiberlike structures called microtubules that play a key role in the cells' life cycle. It produces far fewer of the miserable side effects of platinum drugs.

By now I had become well acquainted with the private wing of Mount Sinai Medical Center called 11-West, where I would go to take my occasional hits of chemo. That part of the hospital should be named Mount Sinai Hotel: There's a paneled reception area with fresh flowers; rooms are furnished with faux Early American chairs and fruit-print draperies; rolling tables in the halls bear the remnants of room service dinners. I was able to keep the chemo nurse I'd had all along, Ann Bush—there's something about the stability of medical personnel that feeds your sense of security and well-being. The staff knew that I liked to watch videos to pass the time, so when I'd arrive there were sign-up sheets ready for me to choose, and they knew I wanted my bill settled that night so I could escape early the next morning and go to work. With all their formalities, hospitals will run you into the ground if you let them, and when you're a frequent flier, you have to be sure that you run *them*. If my chemo was not ready when I arrived, I wanted to know why. I'd get aggressive about it too. I'd call the pharmacy, and I wouldn't take any bullshit. One time when Ann was away, the system broke down and I had to wait from noon until eight P.M. for my medicine. I read them the riot act. A little delay I could understand, but eight hours? I don't think so. I'm ill, I'm busy, and I'm paying.

It was typical of Andrew, during all of this, to always look for ways to divert my attention. He desperately wanted to have a twenty-fifth wedding anniversary bash. We had promised ourselves that, if we made it this far, New Orleans blues and jazz legend Dr. John would play at our party—our present to ourselves. Held at our house in East Hampton, the party had a wonderful, casual, summer feel: no speeches, hundreds of lobsters, Chinese lanterns bobbing in the breeze. Friends and family had traveled from England for the party: Mummy, Lois, and my best friend, Libby, whom I'd known since I was eleven, and her husband. From the city, my staff arrived with spouses, boyfriends, and children, and mingled with my fashion friends from the Hamptons: Carrie Donovan; Donna Karan, who ate six lobsters; Isaac Mizrahi; Nicole Miller, her husband, and new baby. Of course, Grace Coddington and Didier Malige were there, as were my friends Terry and Joanie McDonell (the editor of *Men's Journal* and his author wife). Andrew and I danced all night with the likes of Richard Gere, Carey Lowell, and Dominick and Griffin Dunne, I hardly remember eating, and the spirit of the gathering was one of friendship and hope.

By September I was becoming sick and tired of Taxol. It was having little effect on my CA-125 and seemed to be making no difference in making me better. It didn't make me throw up, but I felt absolutely beaten down, just wrung out and hung up to dry. One afternoon, the Princess of Wales called me and I started to moan about my plight. She became strong and protective and said, "Liz, it's your life, it's your body. If you don't want any more chemo, just tell the doctors to stop. You have to be in control." That was all I needed. Dr. Dottino agreed to stop the treatment, and I began to thrive, with my hair growing back in a very spiky fashion. Repeated CAT scans were stable. Then at the beginning of December 1996, a lump about the size of a fifty-cent piece appeared on my neck. I wasn't too concerned—for one thing, it got smaller and smaller until it became the size of a dime, and for another, I've always had a lump on my back that's been poked by various doctors and pronounced a perfectly normal but gristly piece of spine. Even Dottino didn't act like it was a big deal—it could have been swollen glands from the sort of winter bug that was felling half of New York. And I really had no time for new worries—I was preparing to host the party of the year.

I had agreed to cochair the annual benefit for the Costume Institute at the Metropolitan Museum of Art, and I could have used a clone. LVMH, the French luxury-goods conglomerate that owns Louis Vuitton luggage, Moët & Chandon champagne, Hennessy cognac, and Christian Dior, was sponsoring the gala that year in honor of Dior's fiftieth anniversary. It was actually Carmel Snow, then editor-in-chief of *Harper's Bazaar*, whose compliment about Dior's collection in 1947 became an enduring term: "It's quite a revolution, dear Christian. Your dresses have such a new look." The situation was delicate because Gianfranco Ferré, the bearded, bearish Italian designer for the grand and very French House of Dior, was being replaced by the brilliant British designer John Galliano, but Ferré was nonetheless assigned the departing task of helping to conceptualize the decoration of the Great Hall, at the entrance of the Metropolitan.

The Costume Institute owns quite a few Diors, but when any clothes owned by the museum are displayed, they have to be encased in glass, and I wanted people to really *see* them, to walk in and know immediately they were celebrating fashion. So we borrowed dozens and dozens of amazing creations from private clients: the dresses that took Olivia de Havilland and Leslie Caron to the Academy Awards; the black-and-silver crepe Sophia Loren wore in *Arabesque*; the black-and-cream silk Ingrid Bergman wore in *Indiscreet*, lent by Isabella Rossellini. We had a blue damask from Isabelle Adjani and a floral organza from Tina Turner (who said that when she wore it, men kept coming up and asking if they could water her).

Extraordinary logistics and orchestrations and machinations were involved in acquiring all these clothes, and I had help in particular from Jane Cattani, *Bazaar*'s European editor, who performed miracles of coordination in bringing Eva Peron's Dior dresses out of the Argentinian archives with the gracious help of Eva's niece, Maria-Cristina Alvarez Rodriguez Alvesi. The dresses were to be prominently displayed on invisible structures, to look as though they were suspended in thin air, on top of round platforms in the Great Hall which guests could admire while standing or while lounging on sumptuous sofas that were covered with signature Dior gray-and-white stripes. *And* we had exactly one day to set everything up: The museum closed on Sunday at five P.M., and the party was Monday night.

The Princess of Wales was coming from London with her sister Lady Sarah McCorquodale, just for the night. I had their suite at the Carlyle filled with flowers and candles, along with T-shirts and skateboarding magazines as souvenirs for Diana's sons, since she wouldn't have time to shop. I met them at the airport, where there was a helicopter waiting to bring us into Manhattan, and I escorted them to the hotel before rushing home to dress. I was wearing the last Gianfranco Ferré made for Dior, and the princess was wearing the first John Galliano, both navy blue. Diana had problems keeping the lace straps of her dress up and said that Prince William would have been horrified if he had seen the bareness of the gown. She looked wonderful. But you can't please everybody: Mickey Drexler, president of The Gap, Inc., happened to be waiting in the hotel lobby with his young daughter, and she was disappointed that the princess wasn't wearing a crown.

It's painful now to recall the clamor of attention she received, since it was the same kind of obsession with her every move that led to her death. By the time I returned to the Carlyle to collect her, there was already a crowd gathered outside. Andrew and I had to run the gauntlet of paparazzi and nearly got shut out from the limousine in the crush. As we were pulling away from the curb, a man banged on window.

"Can I have an autograph?" he shouted through the glass.

"I'll have to do it when I get back," Diana said with a smile. But he wouldn't give up. Running behind the car, he followed us around the block, and when we stopped at a traffic light, he was at the window again.

"Should I get out and deal with him?" Andrew asked. But we were just a few blocks from the museum, and the fan gave up the chase as our car picked up speed.

With Andrew functioning as bodyguard (even though we had security surrounding us at all times), long-legged Diana shot up the grand steps with me struggling to keep pace. The sheer volume of the photographers shouting, "Diana, Diana," a million times over, and the blinding flash of the cameras, gave me a brief and terrifying taste of what the princess faced almost every day of her life. Film footage of our arrival that night played across the world the following day. In very different circumstances, it was endlessly reprised in the days after her death.

Greeting us at the top of the stairs as we entered the museum were Bernard Arnault and his wife Hélène, and designer Christian Lacroix. Other special guests that evening included Madame Chirac, wife of the French president, and Madame Pompidou, as well as many important stars from or related to the fashion world: John Mellencamp and his wife, model Elaine Irwin; Calvin Klein with Christy Turlington as his date; Linda Evangelista and Kyle MacLachlan, and Donna Karan with her husband, Stephan Weiss.

The princess looked so stunning that the assembled guests were intimidated. This is such a traditionally glamorous night in New York—it's the gala to end all galas. The richest, most elegant New Yorkers pull out every stop, donning magnificent dresses and enormous jewels. But very few actually approached Diana to say hello. In retrospect, I wish that I had organized a small salon off to the side where people could come a few at a time, in order to give everyone a chance to meet her.

There were almost 900 guests seated for dinner in the museum's main dining hall, which had been decorated to look like Paris's Avenue Montaigne in the spring, complete with a soundtrack of petits oiseaux chirping. The princess sat between Bernard Arnault and John Galliano. I was on John's other side, ready to stem the flow of well-wishers heading toward Diana.

The menu had been created by a French caterer who had flown in for the evening to oversee the preparation of each plate. The House of Dior had designed beautiful green and white organza table linens and a limited-edition china pattern for the evening using its signature flower, lily-of-the-valley. We were shocked to see the matching embroidered napkins being swiped off the table before the last of the tarte des demoiselles tatin and green apple sorbet had been consumed. Here I was, surrounded by the elite of

263

New York society, and there they were, stealing! I think Martha Stewart made off with a set of six!

AFTER DINNER, THE guests at my table accompanied Diana out of the dining room, following the most secretive of routes. From the second-floor balcony she stopped to peer out over the growing fashion crowd of 2,000 who had assembled for the after-dinner party. (Andrew was busy pointing out all the transvestites!) We continued toward the car, with Diana taking a moment to observe the crowd one more time before departing. I'll never forget that moment. She looked every inch the princess ... even without a crown.

After seeing her safely to her car, I made my way back to the Temple of Dendur to join the massive crowd of kids. Our entertainer for the evening, Maxi Priest and his band, were in full swing, and the room was awesome, with images of Dior's work projected on the walls. As part of the event, we had organized a "Design Your Own Dior" contest, which was judged throughout the evening. The winner's dress was a modern take on the New Look, made out of signature Dior-gray colored paper, and a hat topped off with a Dior perfume box—very creative! The evening had been a marked success. Relieved and satisfied, Andrew and I had a glass of champagne and danced into the small hours.

THE NEXT MORNING, still wobbly from champagne, I got a call from my chemo nurse, Ann Bush, who said she'd been trying to reach me, only realizing that I'd been otherwise occupied when she saw the TV coverage of the Met dinner. I had a problem: My latest CA-125 count was 10,000.

"I should be dead," I said.

"You certainly shouldn't be dancing in the Temple of Dendur," she replied. It turns out that the number on a CA-125 test doesn't correlate to the amount of disease—my score of 10,000 was really no more significant than if it had been 1,000, and when I was retested it went down to 500—but it did mean there was cancer somewhere. I needed another CAT scan, and the lump on my neck was to be scanned too. Andrew's response was "Shit." We'd both learned not to panic or overreact, not to try cheering each other with false bromides, but simply to proceed as calmly as possible to the next step. En route to the airport with the princess, I confided in her and got a big, comforting hug, but I didn't tell anyone else.

The scan confirmed that, yes, the lump on my neck was a very small mass and Dottino felt it should come out and be biopsied. It would be a minor procedure, scheduled for the following Wednesday. But that Tuesday was the *Bazaar* Christmas party at a smart new restaurant called Patroon. I seemed to be specializing in putting on a cheerful countenance for parties the night before surgery. But I was cheerful. I do not go into calamity mode about ominous possibilities. I deal with what I have to deal with when I have to deal with it.

The next morning, Dottino came to get me in the ambulatory surgery unit, took me by the hand, and walked me into the OR. The whole procedure lasted about twenty minutes, and I was home by lunch. The lump turned out to be ovarian cancer. The doctor said that when he put a biopsy slide of my original tumor next to a slide of this one, they looked identical. That the lump had got so much smaller all on its own was an extremely good sign: It meant that my body must have been mounting some kind of response—not eradicating cancer, but keeping it in check. I agreed to do some more chemotherapy as a precaution in early 1997, but only after the couture shows in Paris. It is with mock consternation that Dottino complains everything with me is a negotiation.

I know people were commenting that I looked unwell, and I tried to explain my malaise as an extended repercussion of treatment, but I see photographs of myself from that time and realize I probably wasn't fooling anyone. I didn't want to concede publicly that despite my strength of will, cancer was still thumbing its nose at me, and I didn't want to disappoint people who'd been rooting for my victory. I needed time to adjust my own head to the idea of *living* with cancer, just as others live with HIV, diabetes, or high blood pressure.

I found it heartening recently to read in the *Conversations* newsletter the stories of fifty long-term survivors of ovarian cancer: a woman in Cleveland, Ohio, who is twenty-two years past diagnosis with ten different remissions and recurrences; a woman in Miami, Florida, who has been cancer-free for ten years after stage IV disease; a woman in Corpus Christi, Texas, whose six-pound tumor was removed eight years ago; a woman in Knoxville, Tennessee, who has survived five years with ovarian cancer and fifteen years with breast cancer. The overwhelming message of such a roll call is: You can beat this, or at least you can live with it. "There are no guarantees," says Dottino cautiously. "With some patients, the cancer still comes back. Maybe it's genetic, and we can't change genetics. That's why gene therapy is the hope of the future. Right now we just put out isolated fires." Out of the fourteen women who were included with me in the protocol for bone marrow transplant, one died from the assault of BMT, and there has been a recurrence of cancer in all but one of the others. Ovarian cancer is Hercules, Paul Bunyan, and Arnold Schwarzenegger rolled into one, a vigorous and stalwart opponent. It comes back. But some women contract a variety of ovarian cancer so virulent that they are dead within eighteen months, despite all intervention, while I and others live with ovarian cancer as if it's a chronic disease, periodically getting treated. As more time passes, access to new drugs increases, offering greater hope and longer life.

Peter Dottino says I seem to be moving in that direction. I know I'm an extremely healthy person, even though I have cancer. Last winter we went skiing in Snowmass, and I did a dozen runs every day while the men in my family played around with snowshoes and snowboards. (Wimps!) The ground has been shaken under all of us, but my sons are beginning to assimilate my "Timex" status ("takes a licking and keeps on ticking") in their lives. We got a wary call from one of Christopher's teachers when his class was

266

assigned to do reports about their parents, and Chris said matter-of-factly, "My mother's having chemo." I think that exposure to serious illness has given the boys a capacity for compassion not usually seen at their age. One day Robbie told me that the mother of one of his friends had been diagnosed with breast cancer. "Can she talk to you about it?" he asked.

"Yes, of course," I replied, "but I don't have breast cancer."

"I know, I know, I know," he said, a little annoyed at my obtuseness. "But it's *cancer*." He understood that the ground was shaking under his friend's family too and wanted to help.

Last year Chris was making a Christmas "wish list" for the family, a custom I remember from my own childhood, with prohibitions against material goods. For Andrew he wished success with his ingenious new exercise device. For Robbie he wished admission to his first-choice prep school. I wondered what he was going to wish for me, hoping it would not reflect any repressed concerns about my health. It turned out to be a wish that Mummy's magazine would go on succeeding forever. He seemed to take it for granted *I* would.

Ironically, there is no "standard of care" for where I am now. That's because, until recently, women with ovarian cancer died before they reached this point. The treatment for women like me is quite individualized, which is why I started consulting Dr. Robert Nagourney of Rational Therapeutics in Long Beach, California. I found Dr. Nagourney quite by chance—my assistant Stephanie Albertson was watching *Hard Copy* and they happened to run an ovarian cancer piece, featuring Nagourney, which she taped for me. We sent the tape to Dr. Dottino, who recognized Nagourney as a medical school colleague and immediately contacted him. Nagourney is a classically trained physician who has become a self-described contrarian in the field of cancer research. "Almost everything you know about human cancer is wrong," he says defiantly. "If I asked you what makes a cancer cell different, you'd say it divides too rapidly. Wrong. Cancer cells do not grow too much, they die too little. We've been developing drugs that stop cells from growing, but cancers learn how to remain alive. They're not having quintuplets, but they're continuing to have offspring into their hundredth year."

Drugs that may kill cancer cells in the test tube fail in human beings because of this wrongheaded "birth control" approach, according to Nagourney. "What happens when you give those drugs to patients?" he asks. "All the cells in the body that grow normally, like the bone marrow and the hair and the gut, get injured, and at the end of the day the only thing that doesn't get injured is the tumor. Cancer therapy is brutal; it's felonious assault. And the survival of ovarian cancer in the last twenty years has only budged a few percent, so we are not much further ahead. Thank you very much, National Cancer Institute, you're all fired."

Nagourney says that facing a danger like cancer is the same as confronting a bank robber: "Do you step up to the thief and suggest that he use a condom so your grandchildren will not be confronting his grandchildren, or do you put a bullet between his eyes? That's what you're dealing with in cancer medicine. You want to come up with bullets, not birth control. We have a collection of birth-control pills. Sometimes one of the tumors will choke on the pills and die, when you raise the dose up so high it's like dumping a truckload on your head: That's called a bone marrow transplant. You have successfully crushed the cancer, but incidentally it might have been easier to do it another way. Yes, you can get from San Francisco to Los Angeles via Cincinnati, but there's a route along the Pacific Coast that will get you there in five hours, not five days."

The growth and death of cells in the human body sounds almost like Greek tragedy, as Nagourney describes it. "Cells grow all the time," he says. "Your body is replacing itself every instant—just sitting there, you've made about ten million red blood cells. But in order to replace itself, the body kills off the father or mother cell and carries on with the child. And three months later, it kills off that child and carries on with its offspring." The finite life and programmed death of a cell is called apoptosis, and when one of the seventy or eighty different chemotherapy drugs now in use actually works, according to Nagourney, it is because the drug has fostered apoptosis, triggering the cancer cell's escape clause. "Cisplatin turns out to be a classic inducer of apoptosis. If a drug can induce apoptosis in a test tube, it has the capacity to help the patient. So what I am doing today is seeking out that fraction of the American cancer population for whom the available crummy drugs work. That's the best I can do, making the best of a bad situation. What I'd *like* to do is to use my understanding of and insights into cancer biology to develop some meaningful drugs. Wouldn't that be fun?"

At his lab, housed in a modest one-story building on a quiet residential street, Nagourney provides a service that should be available to every cancer patient: He gets a sample of the malignant tissue, shipped by overnight courier, and tests its response to dozens and dozens of different chemotherapy cocktails, sometimes coming up with unorthodox recommendations—perhaps a drug traditionally used against lymphoma that seems effective against liver cancer, or an older drug that works better than a more recent incarnation. Taxol and cisplatin may be the gold standard for advanced ovarian cancer, but my particular type wasn't told the rules: It's *resistant* to Taxol. And despite the fact that it has waged prior battles with cisplatin, my cancer is still sensitive to that drug, also to Navelbine, a drug usually used against lung cancer, and Topotecan, a new drug that prohibits the growth of tumors by suppressing an enzyme essential in replicating DNA. The trick is always to kill the malignant cells without sacrificing too many of the cells that sustain life. "There are all kinds of things that will induce cancer cells' death," says Nagourney. "I could kill your cancer by simply injecting bleach into your veins, but you'd be dead in an instant."

THERE'S A TERRIBLE unfairness to cancer, beyond the fact of the disease itself: You're given a life-threatening diagnosis, and your mind is numb, but you *must* make some decisions that will determine whether you live or die. You must become a good consumer,

269

just as if you were choosing a car or refrigerator. It's not *First, You Cry* but first, you buy, and what you're shopping for is the finest medicine available. A recent study of patients in more than 900 U.S. hospitals showed that the chance of surviving ovarian cancer is directly related to the type of doctor who operates: The best survival rate is with a gynecological oncologist; second-best is with an ob/gyn; third-best with a general surgeon. Let the obstetricians deliver babies, and let the general surgeons remove gall bladders— when you have ovarian cancer, you do not want second- or third-best. If your doctor says you're going to get "standard of care" treatment, maybe that's not good enough. Maybe you want to call the National Cancer Institute and get a list of research trials going on at medical centers all over the country, where you will get *at least* the standard of care and also some new, auspicious tweaking of the standard. That's how progress takes place in medicine: People like you and me participate in promising but still unproven treatments. We further the cause of science at the same time that we improve our own chances.

The minute I stop writing this book, new research will come along that will make my message dated, if not obsolete. But there is still not enough money given to research. While breast cancer has become the darling of the fashion and beauty industries— Avon, Estée Lauder, Danskin, Lee Jeans, and New Balance Shoes have all become part of the breast cancer crusade—and it is an undeniably worthy cause, ovarian cancer is still something of a Cinderella. There are no pink ribbons for this disease, no postage stamp. Our support trickles in. It's wonderful that the Italian Federation of Shoe Manufacturers wants to sponsor a dinner and hand me a $40,000 check for research. But where are our American champions?

I'm trying to bring ovarian cancer into the public vocabulary. Recently I heard the radio personality Howard Stern talk about making the movie of his book *Private Parts*. The director, Betty Thomas, was trying to capture a certain expression of shock on Stern's face that she couldn't seem to elicit. So, off camera, the director went up to him and said, "I have something to tell you: I

270

have ovarian cancer." Stern's face froze in stunned surprise, and the director said, "*That's* the look I want." Strange as it may sound, I was excited when I heard this story. The director could have chosen any number of jolting words, but she picked "ovarian cancer." It's entering the common parlance. If we're ever going to conquer it, we've got to get people talking about it.

It is unlikely that you will ever have ovarian cancer, and you should not go through life worrying about it. But if you are experiencing any of the warning signs, if you're making the rounds of gastroenterologists or X-ray technicians or even psychiatrists to diagnose persistent abdominal distress, ask about a CA-125 blood test and a transvaginal ultrasound. Do not let lack of awareness— yours or the professionals'—thwart your chance to pounce on an early, *curable* disease.

In the summer of 1997, I was hooked up once again to an IV tube dripping cancer-fighting drugs into my veins. My CA-125 is a roller coaster: It goes up, I get some chemo, and then it goes down. Chemo is my least favorite thing to do in life, and I hope to continue doing it for another fifty years. I'm planning to be around for a long time, and I am determined to lie in a shallow grave—no room for other unwitting victims of this miserable disease.

The day I was to have my first treatment with the new chemo-therapy drug called Topotecan, July 15, 1997, I learned that my friend Gianni Versace, who was the same age as myself, had been tragically and meaninglessly gunned down outside his home in Miami Beach. I had seen him just a week before, at a festive dinner at the Ritz in Paris after his couture show, when we shared a chair, one cheek each, to laugh and gab and celebrate. It was Gianni who practically invented the modern fashion show, infusing it with powerful imagery and blasting rock soundtracks, front-row cel-ebrities, name-brand models, the glitz and seductiveness of bold, decadent, unabashedly sexual clothes. He had just come through his own bout with a rare cancer of the ear, opting to have radiation treatment in lieu of surgery, which might have caused distortion in the muscles of his vibrant, handsome face, and we had talked about the fragility of life, the drama of facing one's own mortality. The Topotecan treatment was so noninvasive that I found myself able to respond by phone to requests for interviews about Gianni that afternoon. Being called upon to eulogize him on *Good Morning America* and *Charlie Rose* the same week I was fighting my own continuing skirmish crystallized for me the need to savor every moment of life.

And then, just weeks later, I was grieving for another friend. I learned that a car carrying the Princess of Wales had crashed in a Paris tunnel much the way millions of others heard the news: watching TV at home on the Saturday night of a long Labor Day weekend. The first bulletins reported the death of her companion, Dodi Fayed, but indicated only that Diana had been injured. Horrified but still hopeful, Andrew and I stayed close to CNN for several hours, mindlessly and endlessly repeating to ourselves the words "It can't have happened"—until we both fell into a stunned sleep. When the phone rang around midnight, there was a moment between the registering of its shrill ring and wakefulness that I realized it couldn't be good news. The caller was Veronica Hearst, confirming Diana's death, and then there were no words, profane or otherwise, only tears.

The phone became an enemy for the next week. In the wee hours of that first morning, an MCI operator called to say that television reporter Willow Bay (who didn't have our unlisted number) was requesting to be put through on an "emergency" basis. (The emergency was the need to get a comment for the Sunday edition of *Good Morning America*. Andrew declined in terms that could not be repeated on a family broadcast.) Both ABC and NBC had camera crews ready in the Hamptons to interview people. I declined everything, apart from one phone interview with Barbara Walters when I was still in a state of shock, and by the time I returned to my office on Tuesday, there were sixty-three requests for interviews. By Friday, when I left for the funeral, the count was over a hundred. Despite feeling numb and devastated, I ended up making a few carefully selected comments, resigning myself to the insatiable demand for information and remembrances. Before the cameras started rolling for an interview with Dan Rather in London after the funeral, he leaned forward somewhat conspiratorially. "To give you an idea of the kind of pressure we're under," he said, "I was told to ask you what you thought the princess would be wearing in her coffin, but I won't."

Patrick Demarchelier and I flew together to London, and the shrine of flowers left by the public was visible from the air as the plane broke through the clouds. I had asked a London florist, Evelyn Shearer from Pulbrook and Gould, whom I had always used for bouquets for Diana's birthday, to arrange for an armload of white lilies to be waiting in the car that picked us up at Heathrow Airport. I had asked the princess's butler, Paul Burrell, if I could bring them to her home in Kensington Palace, where her coffin was to rest that Friday night. It was 5:58 P.M. when we got in the car, and Queen Elizabeth was addressing the nation at 6, so we listened to her words on the radio. It was an astonishing break with tradition for the monarchy to respond to the public in this way, but she was still remote, unemotional, using words like "admire" and "respect" in lieu of any expressions of affection.

When I arrived at Kensington Palace I gave my name to a policeman at the gate and took the lilies to a private garden near her apartments. You could smell the floral alms in the public part of the park before you could see them, a cloying insistence, like too much perfume, and the trees were strewn with teddy bears, poems, candles, photographs. We stayed in the park for an hour. As I was helping a little girl balance on a police barrier so she could see over the crowd to the swarm of tributes, her father told me that Mother Teresa had died. The news spread through the crowd, yet for all the hundreds of people there, it was amazingly quiet. The entrances into the park were so choked with people that we had to exit onto the street through a public men's room—it didn't please the policeman on duty, but he finally said, "I don't think I can stop you, ma'am."

The hairdresser Sam McKnight and I had planned dinner that night at San Lorenzo. It was to be a comfort session for the princess's photographic team. Mary Greenwell, who so often did the princess's makeup, was there. Patrick Demarchelier came too, and Anna Harvey flew down from her holiday in Scotland to join us. Mara, the owner of San Lorenzo, was a great friend of the princess, and so we all had much to remember, and much to cry about. But it was as therapeutic as we'd wanted it to be—there was even some laughter at good times remembered.

The next morning, Saturday, September 6, it felt as if London had been hit by a neutron bomb—the streets were empty (except for the cortege route), and eerily silent (except for the buzz of police helicopters overhead). Invitations to the funeral had been issued by the Lord Chamberlain based on Diana's Christmas card list, and holding my simple entrance card, I realized that my ticket would be the last contact from Diana to be placed in the walnut box on my desk at home containing all her cards and letters. As I rode down Park Lane, a Rolls-Royce pulled away from the Dorchester Hotel, and I waved to Donatella and Santo Versace, who'd buried their brother so few weeks before. In the queue to enter Westminster Abbey, I was next to John Galliano, Bernard Arnault, and some nuns—a wonderful commentary on Diana's vast scope of influence and friendship.

Patrick Demarchelier and I were seated in the first row of the first nave, and when the coffin was brought in, covered with the maroon and gold royal standard and borne by red-coated Welsh Guards with interlocked arms, I simply broke down. But as sometimes happens in deeply moving moments, an inappropriate thought popped into my head. The eight Welsh guards were sweating under the weight of the lead-lined coffin, and I thought how amused the princess would have been, making eight beefy men suffer under her weight. As the funeral ended, Karl Lagerfeld, Amanda Harlech, Patrick, and I were among the last to exit the Abbey. We seemed reluctant to leave the memories behind. On a whim, we decided to go to the Ritz for lunch, thinking that Diana would enjoy the idea of being remembered in London's most beautiful dining room. We tried not to be funereal—Diana wouldn't have liked that—and we were all struck by how amazing it was to have seen the entire royal family file past us, with all the teenagers that we remembered as babies, and we all remarked on how good Princess Anne's legs were. But mostly, we remembered Diana.

One day in early August, the princess had left a telephone message saying, "I'm sorry to not have called, but I'm a bit evasive at the moment." I think she must have meant elusive. I do hope she had a wonderful time in those "evasive" last weeks of her life. I've no wish to canonize her. It was her *un*saintliness, her "common touch," her all-too-familiar and less-than-regal problems that made people respond to her as they did. The papers called her a good soldier, and her brother, Earl Spencer, spoke eloquently of her innermost feelings of suffering and unworthiness, "her constituency of the rejected." She talked about things only in oblique references, seldom drawing attention to the fractured fairy tale of her existence. She was the "very British girl," as Earl Spencer called her, who married the Prince Charming *every* British girl wanted to marry—my father had wanted *me* to marry him—and then the bubble had burst.

I always observed propriety with the princess, never overstepping the boundaries of warm but respectful friendship or giving voice to the curiosity of journalism. I chatted with her about her anger and resentment at being stripped of "HRH," her royal honorific, and her indignation at having to forfeit the eventual title of Queen. And I know she worried that since she no longer had official status, the clout that she brought to her work for good causes would decrease. I talked to her about "white light," after my own experience with rising platelets so closely paralleled the palliative effect I saw in the sick and disabled people she touched. She knew she had healing powers, not in the literal sense of eradicating illness but a transference of strength and tenderness.

She talked to me of her desire for her sons to know about people's insecurities and stresses, their hopes and dreams. Diana drew so much from being a mother. That was her first job. When you talked to her, the second sentence was always about the children. Sometimes I'd ring up and say, "What's that noise?" and she'd be sitting on the bed with the boys watching some terrible

275

kung-fu video they wanted to see. When Harry and William first started at boarding school, she talked about how it killed her to leave them there. She was particularly worried about William at Eton being hounded by the press and whether he could handle it. She was trying hard to teach her sons how to cope with press attention, and to accept that it was something they were going to have to live with. William saw how reporters and photographers treated her. He understood her fury with them, and he also understood that she courted them from time to time. William was very close to his mother and was full of sympathy for her. He wanted her to be happy and he knew she had gone through a lot of unhappiness, and that the media had contributed to that.

Diana was stoic about her situation after the divorce. It used to upset me sometimes that she couldn't be with her children on some of the most important occasions. She rang me on Christmas Day 1996 just to see how I was. And I felt so guilty—there I was, sitting in my house in the country with my kids, and when I asked her if she was with hers, she said, "Oh no, they're in Scotland shooting little furry things with their father." She didn't have a trace of bitterness. She knew she had to bow to the rules of the court, and she was being very strong about it.

Because the princess and I had sons about the same age, the worst part of her death for me is thinking of those boys without her. I dearly hope that their father and family and friends will not, as Earl Spencer said in his eulogy, consign them strictly to onerous duty and tradition, but will remember their mother's insistence that their lives include myriad experiences, from soul-enriching encounters with the downtrodden of society to the fun of fast-food hamburgers and amusement-park rides. At the funeral, as the two young princes followed their mother's coffin, I caught William's eye for an instant, and I felt the anguish of a mother's unfinished business—real and final for Diana, implied and feared for a cancer survivor like me. All the dread and foreboding of those first moments after my diagnosis came flooding back, all that a mother who dies too soon misses, all the motherlove her children will never receive.

Not being a religious person, the only message I can take away from the violent and premature loss of such dear friends, and from facing my own mortality, is: Carpe diem. Seize the day. Diana and Gianni, two vibrant human beings in the prime of life, are gone, and I am thriving. If anything, I had imagined the princess attending *my* memorial service, and here I was, attending hers. I don't know how to resolve this conundrum, to make peace with these ridiculous facts, except to embrace the long life that she was denied.

# epilogue

I NEVER WANTED to be a poster girl for cancer. But cancer has become part of who I am, along with my big feet and my English accent. I am five feet seven, I have greenish eyes, I was born on September 7 (the same day as Queen Elizabeth I), and I have ovarian cancer. So do almost 175,000 other women in the United States. A lot of them write to me, from all over the country, often addressing me as "Liz"—there is a camaraderie about a shared experience that seems to supersede formalities and decorum—and their letters are full of compassion, anger, and hope. A woman in Deatsville, Alabama, addressed me as "Dear Liz, My Sister." A woman in Boulder, Colorado, wrote that two fertility specialists had recommended Clomid, and when she specifically asked about the risk of cancer, she was told not to worry. (The second doctor prescribed it over the phone, never having met her.) A woman in Lubbock, Texas, now designs furniture for cancer treatment centers. And my hospital neighbor during the isolation of bone marrow transplant—the woman who hallucinated about the nurses having hashish parties in her room—wrote that those drugs were better than anything she had in the 1960s.

But it's the newly diagnosed women who touch me the most. I remember the emotions described in these letters. They're the feelings I had during chemotherapy, when I would sit at home making photo albums for my sons, in case I wasn't going to be around much longer. Those feelings have changed. If fighting

278

cancer means going to war, then I'm there. Like a samurai strategist, I keep my friends close and my enemies closer. I don't run away from cancer. I study it, anticipate it, confront it, wrestle with it. But you'd be surprised how little time I spend thinking about it. I do not feel desperate; I have found the best doctors and entrusted myself to their care, their wisdom, their energy, and their medicine.

Every woman in a similar position has to decide for herself how to live so that she doesn't feel like there is an anvil hanging over her head. For me it means maintaining normalcy, coming to work each day because I'm in charge. And it means being a mom, because moms aren't sick. My kids will tease, "You're not going to dive in the pool," and I say, "Watch me." I live in my noisy, messy household of men with too much sports on TV, and the toilet seats forever up, and nobody even noticing the newly cleaned curtains in the dining room. And I wouldn't have it any other way. Andrew and I drove Robbie to boarding school last fall with the typical parents' mixed emotions about the firstborn leaving the nest. I could have resisted this move, keeping him close to home, fearful that each year with him might be my last. Instead, I choose to be grateful for each year and to believe that there will be plenty more. It's a decision I make, like other executive decisions. And so far, I'm winning.

I've also reached some decisions about *how* I will grow old, if I get to grow old. I turned fifty on my last birthday, the day after Princess Diana's funeral. Andrew was insistent that we celebrate, no matter what; we both thought I'd never even make fifty years old. But there I was. I'm wrinkling along with the rest of them, and frankly, I don't care if I develop the face of a shar-pei, and my boobs hit the floor. I'm happy to age with my body. I already have a gallery of scars, and I have no wish to add to the collection.

Whenever I have been in the hospital, many wonderful people have gone to their churches and temples to kneel and light candles and say prayers and direct healing white light to me. I was grateful for every bit of it. When I was having my BMT, one friend asked what she could do, and I suggested that she select a beautiful stone for her garden and think of me whenever she saw it. She went to a place in British Columbia where the Indians draw symbols on stones, and brought back one with a frog painted on it. The day she put it in the garden, a real frog came out of the woods to swim in her pool and leap around the stone. It returned every day to swim until *I* was "out of the woods" and feeling much better. When I had really improved, the frog went back to the forest and never came to swim again.

And that's all I'm trying to do now—keep the frog in the forest.

# resources

AUSTRALIA

**Gynaecological Cancer Counselling**
Westmead Centre for
    Gynaecological Cancer
Westmead Hospital
Westmead NSW 2145
(02) 9845 6712 or (02) 9845 6699

*Gynaecological Oncology*
Royal Hospital for Women
Barker Street
Randwick NSW 2031
(02) 9382 6240

NEW ZEALAND

**Cancer Society of New Zealand (Inc)**
Auckland Division
PO Box 1724
Auckland
(09) 524 2628
0800 800 426 (toll-free)
Provides a network of support
    throughout the country.

SOUTH AFRICA

**Cancer Association of South Africa**
(Gauteng Region)
1 Saxonwold Drive

Saxonwold 2196
South Africa
27 11 646 5628
Fax: 27 11 646 2914

UNITED KINGDOM

**Action Cancer**
1 Marlborough Park
Belfast BT9 6XS
01232 661081
Fax: 01232 683931
Provides screening, information,
    advice and counselling.

**The Anthony Nolan Bone Marrow
    Trust**
The Royal Free Hospital
Pond Street
Hampstead
London NW3 2QG
0171 284 1234
Fax: 0171 284 8226
Donor Hotline: 0990 111533
Fundraising Enquiries: 0990 111517
Undertakes research and has
    established a register of over
    280,000 potential bone marrow
    donors for patients including
    those with cancer.

**BACUP**
*See* CancerBACUP

**British Association for Counselling**
1 Regent Place
Rugby
Warwickshire CV21 2PJ
01788 578328
Provides support, protection, and
  information.

**Bristol Cancer Help Centre**
Grove House
Cornwallis Grove
Clifton
Bristol BS8 4PG
0117 980 9505
Offers a healing program that is
  complementary to medical
  treatment.

**CancerBACUP (*formerly known as
  BACUP*)**
3 Bath Place
Rivington Street
London EC2A 3JR
0800 18 11 99
(Glasgow): 0141 553 1553
http://www.cancerbacup.org.uk
Provides information, counselling
  and support for people with
  cancer, their families and
  friends. All services are provided
  free of charge and in
  confidence.

**Cancer Care Society**
21 Zetland Road
Redland
Bristol BS6 7AH
0117 942 7419
Provides support through a national
  network of branches.

**Cancerlink**
11–21 Northdown Street
London N1 9BN
0800 132905 (Textphone available)
Asian Cancer Information Line:
  0800 590415
Support and information on all
  aspects of cancer. Can put people
  in touch with self-help groups
  throughout the UK, and advises
  on forming new groups.

**Carers National Association**
20–25 Glasshouse Yard
London EC1A 4JS
0345 573369 (Mon-Fri 10 am–
  12 noon & 2–4 pm)
Information and support for people
  caring for relatives and friends.

**Chai–Lifeline Cancer Support and
  Centre For Health**
Norwood House
Harmony Way
off Victoria Road
London NW4 2BZ
0181 202 4567
Fax: 0181 202 2111
E-mail: info@chai-lifeline.org.uk
http://www.chai-lifeline.org.uk
Provides Jewish cancer patients,
  their families and friends with
  support. Complementary
  therapies offered.

**Foresight Association for the
  Promotion of Preconceptual Care**
28 The Paddock
Godalming
Surrey GU7 1XD
01483 427 839
Advises on natural drug-free
  approaches to infertility. In the

first instance, send an SAE.

**Gilda's Club**
c/o Munkenbeck & Marshall
Exmouth House
3 Pine Street
London EC1R 0JH
0171 833 8322
Fax: 0171 837 5416
A free resource for anybody touched
  by cancer.

**Hairline International Alopecia
  Patient's Society**
Lyons Court
1668 High Street
Knowle
West Midlands B93 0LY
01564 775281
Advises on wigs, coping with hair
  loss etc. Send an A4 SAE marking
  top of envelope CHEMO.

**The Hospice Information Service**
St Christopher's Hospice
51–59 Lawrie Park Road
Sydenham
London SE26 6DZ
0181 778 9252
Publishes a directory of hospice and
  palliative care services. For a copy
  or details of local services,
  telephone or send a large SAE
  with three first class stamps.

**Human Fertilisation and
  Embryology Authority** (HFEA)
Paxton House
30 Artillery Lane
London E1 7LS
0171 377 5077
Licences all UK clinics dealing with
  *in vitro* fertilization, donor eggs
  etc. Will supply a list of clinics.

**Hysterectomy Support Network**
3 Lynne Close
Green Street Green
Orpington
Kent BR6 6BS
Enables women (and families or
  partners) to contact former
  hysterectomy patients for
  encouragement, advice and
  support.

**Institute for Complementary
  Medicine**
PO Box 194
London SE16 1QZ
0171 237 5165

**Institute of Trichologists**
PO Box 142
Stevenage
Hertfordshire SG1 5UX
01438 387182
E-mail:
  trichologists@ambernet.co.uk
Supplies lists of practising
  trichologists, plus basic leaflets
  about hair loss and treatments.

**Irish Cancer Society**
5 Northumberland Road
Dublin 4
00 353 800 200 700
E-mail:fundraising@irishcancer.ie
Offers all types of support including
  night nursing and home care
  services.

**ISSUE** (*The National Fertility
  Association*)
114 Lichfield Street
Walsall WS1 0YZ
01922 722888 (Mon–Fri 8 am–
  8 pm)

http://www.issue.co.uk
Patient support group offering
  information, support and advice
  on all matters relating to
  infertility. Free telephone
  counselling.

**Let's Face It**
14 Fallowfield
Yately
Hampshire GU46 6LW
01252 879630
E-mail:mike@lfi.u-net.com
http://www.lfi.u-net.com
Primarily a contact point for people
  with facial disfigurement but also
  helps those with hair loss.

**Look Good . . . Feel Better**
Josaron House
5–7 John Princes Street
London W1M 9HD
0171 495 4755
Fax: 0171 493 8061
The program is a free cancer support
  service for women living with
  cancer. Patients are invited to
  attend beauty workshops where
  they receive professional advice
  and guidance on how to cope
  with emotional and appearance-
  related side effects of their
  treatments.

**Macmillan Cancer Relief**
Anchor House
15–19 Britten Street
London SW3 3TZ
0845 601 6161 (Mon–Fri 9.30 am–
  4.30 pm)
9 Castle Terrace Edinburgh EH1
  2DP
0131 229 3276

Working to improve treatment and
  care of cancer patients and their
  families. Specialist Macmillan
  nurses and doctors. Provides
  information plus grants for
  patients in financial difficulties
  (referral via health professional).

**Marie Curie Cancer Care**
28 Belgrave Square
London SW1X 8QG
0171 235 3325
Fax: 0171 823 2380
E-mail:info@mariecurie.org.uk
http://www.mariecurie.org.uk
Provides practical nursing care at
  home and specialist care through
  its Marie Curie Centres. Services
  are free and available after
  assessment.

**The National Cancer Alliance**
PO Box 579
Oxford OX4 1LB
01865 793566
Fax: 01865 251050
Represents the interests and views
  of cancer patients, carers, health
  professionals and groups affected
  by cancer. Publications available.

**Ovacome**
c/o Shirley Lodge
470 London Road
Slough
Berkshire SL3 8QY
01753 714333
Nationwide support group for all
  those affected by ovarian cancer.

**The Sue Ryder Foundation**
Cavendish
Sudbury

Suffolk
01787 280252
Fax: 01787 280548
Nine Sue Ryder Homes in England
specialize in cancer care. Visiting
nurses also care for patients at
home.

**Tak Tent Cancer Support**
Block C20
Western Court
100 University Place
Glasgow G12 6SQ
0141 211 1932

**Tenovus Cancer Information Service**
The Tenovus Cancer Information
Centre
College Buildings
Courtenay Road
Splott
Cardiff CF1 1SA
0800 526527
Fax: 01222 489919
Provides information and emotional
support for cancer patients and
their families. Drop-in Centre for
one-to-one counselling.

**Trendco**
Sheridan House
114–116 Western Road
Hove BN3 1DD
01273 774977
Fax: 01273 720116
Manufactures wigs especially for
women with complete or partial
hair loss.

**The Ulster Cancer Foundation**
40–42 Eglantine Avenue
Belfast BT9 6DX
01232 663439 (Mon–Fri 9 am–
5 pm)

Provides support and counselling on
many aspects of cancer, including
an Ovarian Cancer Support
Service.

**Well Being**, the charity arm of the
Royal College of Obstetricians
and Gynaecologists
The Health Research Charity for
Women and Babies
27 Sussex Place
Regent's Park
London NW1 4SP
0171 262 5337
A major project is the Well Being
Centre for Ovarian Cancer
Research, set up in 1995.

**Women's Nationwide Cancer
Control Campaign**
Suna House
128–130 Curtain Road
London EC2A 3AR
0171 729 2229 (9.30 am–1.00 pm)
E-mail:wnccc@dial.pipex.com
http://dspace.dial.pipex.com/
town/square/gm40/
Focuses on prevention and
protection against cancer in
women.

USA

**American Cancer Society**
404–320–3333 or
800–ACS–2345 (toll-free)
http://www.cancer.org
Provides referrals to cancer-care
centers and services (such as wigs
free of charge); maintains database
of newspaper and magazine
articles; offers ACS position
papers on treatments and
information about medications.

**American Hair Loss Council**
800–274–8717 (toll-free)
Information for women dealing
with hair loss after chemotherapy.

**American Institute for Cancer
Research**
1759 R Street NW
Washington, D.C. 20009
800–843–8114 (toll-free)
Information about nutrition in the
prevention and treatment of
ovarian cancer.

**American Society for Reproductive
Medicine**
409 12th Street SW
Washington, D.C. 20024–2125
202–863–2439
Information about treatment for
infertility.

**BMT Newsletter**
1985 Spruce Avenue
Highland Park, Illinois 60035
847–831–1913
Fax: 847–831–1943
E-mail:bmtnews@transit.nyser.net
Information about bone marrow
transplants, published six times a
year. Free, with suggested
donation of $20.

**Bone Marrow Transplant Family
Support Network**
P.O. Box 845
Avon, Connecticut 06001
800–826–9376 (toll-free)
Counselling, support, and insurance
information.

**Cancer Care Counselling Line**
800–813–HOPE (toll-free)

Free support to patients and their
families.

**Cancer Information Service**
National Cancer Institute
800–4–CANCER (toll-free)
http://cancernet.nci.nih.gov
Information and list of clinical trials.

**Cancer-L Support Group**
LISTSERV@wvnvm.wvnet.edu
(Subscribe Cancer-L Your Name)

**Cancervive**
6500 Wilshire Boulevard
Los Angeles, California 90048
213–655–3758

**Conversations**
P.O. Box 7948
Amarillo, Texas 79114–7948
806–355–2565
Monthly newsletter for women with
ovarian cancer, with optional pen
pal/phone pal list. Free, with
donations welcome.

**Gilda Radner Familial Ovarian
Cancer Registry**
Roswell Park Cancer Institute
Elm and Carlton Streets
Buffalo, New York 14263
800–OVARIAN (toll-free)
http://rpci.med.buffalo.edu/clinic/
gynonc/grwp/html
Information and support for women
with a family history of ovarian
cancer, staffed by volunteers also
at high risk.

**Hereditary Cancer Institute**
Creighton University
2500 California Plaza

Omaha, Nebraska 68178
800–648–8133 (toll-free)
Clinical evaluation for potential
   participation in research projects
   for women with a family history
   of ovarian cancer.

**Marsha Rivkin Ovarian Cancer
   Research Center**
1221 Madison Street
Seattle, Washington 98104
800–422–4547 (toll-free)
Fax: 407–392–6188
Promotes awareness, detection,
   prevention, and research; staffed
   by ovarian cancer survivors.

**Medical Video Productions**
1846 Craig Park Court
St. Louis, Missouri 63146
800–822–3100 (toll-free)
Video titled "The Beauty of
   Control" offers tips on make up
   and wigs for women fighting
   cancer. Cost is $19.95.

**National Bone Marrow Transplant
   Link**
29209 Northwestern Highway,
   #624
Southfield, Michigan 47304
800–LINK–BMT (toll-free)
Fax: 810–287–0321
Public education, support, advocacy,
   and research.

**National Cancer Survivors Day
   Foundation/**
*Coping Magazine*
2019 North Carothers
Franklin, Tennessee 37064
615–794–3006 (for foundation)
615–790–2400 (for magazine)

E-mail:copingmag@aol.com
Subscription is $18 a year.

**National Coalition for Cancer
   Survivorship**
1010 Wayne Avenue
Silver Spring, Maryland 20910
301–650–8868

**National Infertility Network
   Exchange**
P.O. Box 204
East Meadow, New York 11554
516–794–5772

**National Marrow Donor Program**
3433 Broadway Street NE, Suite 400
Minneapolis, Minnesota 55413
800–MARROW–2 (toll-free)
Fax: 612/627–5877
Congressionally authorized
   network with databank of
   tissue-typed bone marrow donor
   volunteers.

**National Ovarian Cancer Coalition**
P.O. Box 4472
Boca Raton, Florida 33429–4472
888–OVARIAN (toll-free)
Fax: 407–392–6188
http://members.aol.com/
   mind2body/nocc.html
Promotes awareness of and research
   about ovarian cancer throughout
   the general population and the
   medical community.

**Ovar'Coming Together**
c/o Pam Faerber
1255 South 900 E
East Zionsville, Indiana 46077
317–769–5561
Support, networking, and education

for ovarian cancer survivors and for all women regarding early warning signs and risks.

**Ovarian Cancer Awareness Quilt**
1521 West Addison Street
Chicago, Illinois 60613
http://www.qcx.com/cancer/
blocks.htm

**Ovarian Cancer National Alliance**
P.O. Box 33107
Washington, DC 20033–0107
202–452–5910
E-mail: Ovarian@aol.com
An umbrella organization which will work nationally to increase public and professional understanding of ovarian cancer, and to advocate for increased research.

**The Ovarian Cancer Research Fund Inc.**
One Pennsylvania Plaza
New York, New York 10119–0165
212–613–5680
Promotes research, education, and awareness about the diagnosis and treatment of ovarian cancer.

**Ovarian Plus**
P.O. Box 498
Paauilo, Hawaii 96776–0498
808–776–1696
Fax: 808–776–1266
E-mail:csinnex@hawaii.edu
http://www.monitor.com/ovarian
Quarterly newsletter about prevention of gynecological cancers. Subscription: $50.

**Ovarian Problems Discussion Group**
LISTSERV@maelstrom.stjohns.edu
(Subscribe ovarian Your Name)

**OVCA Mind 2 BODY**
http://members.aol.com/
mind2body/mind2body.html

**SHARE**
1501 Broadway, Suite 1720
New York, New York 10036
212–719–12044
http://www.noah.cuny.edu/
providers/share.html
Hotline, support groups, wellness programs, and education meetings.

**Society of Gynecological Oncologists**
401 North Michigan Avenue
Chicago, Illinois 60611
312–644–6610
http://www.sgo.org
Provides physician referrals.

**Tender Loving Care Catalogue**
800–850–9445 (toll-free)
Information about products to deal with hair loss.

**Transplant Recipients International Organization**
1000 16th Street NW, Suite 601
Washington, D.C. 20036
800–TRIO–386 (toll-free)
Information and support for those who have undergone or are awaiting bone marrow transplants; a list of local support groups is offered.